SHEET PAN
KETOGENIC

150 ONE-TRAY RECIPES FOR QUICK AND EASY, LOW-CARB MEALS AND HASSLE-FREE CLEANUP

PAMELA ELLGEN

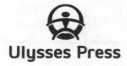

Ulysses Press

Published in the U.S. by
ULYSSES PRESS
P.O. Box 3440
Berkeley, CA 94703
www.ulyssespress.com

5824 4590 7/17

ISBN: 978-1-61243-674-6
Library of Congress Control Number: 2016957550

Printed in the United States by United Graphics Inc.

10 9 8 7 6 5 4 3 2 1

Acquisitions Editor: Casie Vogel
Managing Editor: Claire Chun
Project Editor: Serena Lynn
Editors: Shayna Keyles, Lauren Harrison
Proofreader: Renee Rutledge
Production: Caety Klingman
Front cover design: Michelle Thompson
Cover photographs: Pamela Ellgen

Distributed by Publishers Group West

Contents

INTRODUCTION 1

Chapter One   THE KETOGENIC DIET. 3

Chapter Two   BREAKFAST. 11
Cinnamon Nut Granola 12
Pumpkin Spice Granola. 14
Tropical Coconut Granola. 16
Basic Cloud Bread 18
    Cloud Bread Avocado Toast 19
    Cloud Bread BLT 19
    Cloud Bread Eggs Benedict. 20
Apple Sage Pork Sausage. 21
Savory Breakfast Sausage. 22
Green Shakshuka with Herbs and Za'atar 23
    Traditional Shakshuka 24
Mushroom, Sun-Dried Tomato, and Herb Frittata. 25
Sausage, Rosemary, and Roasted Onion Frittata. 26
Baked Eggs in Avocado 27
    Spicy Harissa Baked Eggs in Avocado 27
    Salmon and Dill Baked Eggs in Avocado. 28
    Bacon and Cheese Baked Eggs in Avocado 28

Chapter Three   SNACKS AND APPETIZERS. .29
Almond Parmesan Crisps. 30
    Vegan Rosemary Hazelnut Crisps. 31
Spiced Mixed Nuts 32
Zucchini Onion Latkes. 33

Garlic and Lemon Roasted Cauliflower............................34
   Roasted Cauliflower with Mint and Pine Nuts..................35
Broiled Romaine Hearts with Roasted Peppers......................36
Smoky Sweet Roasted Cabbage....................................37
Chorizo-Stuffed Mushrooms.......................................38
   Cheesy Artichoke-Stuffed Mushrooms........................39
Asparagus with Hazelnut Romesco................................40
   Roasted Asparagus with Poached Egg.......................41
Prosciutto-Wrapped Asparagus....................................42
Avocado Bacon Fries..43
Fiery Chicken Wings..44
Parmesan Baked Chicken Nuggets.................................45
Crispy Brussels Sprouts and Bacon...............................46
Mesquite Steak and Vegetable Rolls.............................47
Coconut Shrimp...48
Bacon-Wrapped Scallops...49

Chapter Four   VEGETARIAN.....................................50
Spinach and Cheese-Stuffed Portobello Mushrooms................51
Cheesy Spaghetti Squash Bake...................................52
Roasted Red Pepper and Fontina Pizza...........................54
Feta, Olive, and Sun-Dried Tomato Pizza........................56
Four-Cheese Calzone..58
Lasagna Zucchini Boats...60
Kung Pao Cauliflower...61
Roasted Vegetable Frittata.....................................62
   Roasted Fennel and Onion Frittata.........................63
Baked Eggplant Stacks..64
   Vegan Eggplant Stacks with Macadamia Cheese..............65
Broccoli and Tofu Spaghetti Squash Noodle Bowl.................66
Roasted Peppercorn Tofu and Broccolini.........................68
Coconut-Crusted Tofu with Honey Mustard Sauce..................70

Rosemary Pecan Tofu Cutlets. 72

Stuffed Eggplant with Feta and Pine Nuts. 73

Teriyaki Tempeh Skewers. 74

    Barbecue Tempeh with Wilted Spinach. 75

Chapter Five   SEAFOOD. 76

Salsa Verde Shrimp 77

Shrimp Fajita Bowls 78

Prawns Provençal 80

Buttery Lime-Baked Halibut and Scallions. 82

Soy Ginger Salmon with Roasted Mushrooms 84

Baked Salmon with Honey Mustard Cream Sauce 86

Salmon and Fennel with Orange 88

Halibut with Tarragon Compound Butter and Green Beans. 90

Bacon-Wrapped Shrimp 92

Sausage, Shrimp, and Bok Choy 93

Classic Crab Cakes with Lemon Sour Cream 94

Asian Crab Cakes with Sriracha Mayo. 96

Chapter Six   POULTRY. 97

Chicken Chile Relleno. 98

Chicken Enchilada Zucchini Boats 100

Caprese Chicken. 102

Chicken Thighs with Bacon Mustard Cream Sauce 104

Chicken Thighs with Mushrooms and Kale 105

Moroccan Chicken Tagine 106

Broccoli and Chicken Spaghetti Squash Noodle Bowl. 108

Bacon-Wrapped, Guacamole-Stuffed Chicken Breast. 110

Pesto Chicken and Asparagus with Sun-Dried Tomatoes. 111

Smoked Gouda and Butternut Squash Chicken Bake. 112

Cheesy Chicken Fajita Bake. 114

Chicken and Herb-Roasted Vegetables 116

Roasted Chicken Leg Quarters with Bacon and Brussels Sprouts 118

Basic Roasted Chicken. 120

Smoky Garlic Butter Whole Roasted Chicken and Spinach 122

Whole Roasted Chicken with Zucchini, Onions, and Carrots 124

Sausage, Fennel, and Chicken Drumsticks. 126

Chapter Seven PORK 127

Pork Marsala. 128

Prosciutto and Gouda–Stuffed Pork. 130

Slow-Roasted Barbecue Ribs. 132

Citrus and Herb Marinated Pork Shoulder 134

Rainbow Peppercorn Pork Chops with Endive 136

Pork Tenderloin with Radishes and Olive Mayo 138

Smoky Pork Tenderloin with Crispy Cabbage 140

Italian Meatballs. 142

Ham in Tomato Cream Sauce. 143

Vietnamese Pork Meatball Lettuce Wraps 144

Hawaiian Pizza with Cauliflower Crust. 146

Sausage Pizza with Cauliflower Crust 148

Broccoli, Ham, and Mozzarella Bake. 150

Chapter Eight BEEF AND LAMB. 151

Flatiron Steaks with Creamed Spinach 152

Bacon-Wrapped Filet Mignon 154

Chinese Beef and Broccoli 155

Coffee-Crusted Rib Eye Steak. 156

Rib Eye Steaks with Romesco and Roasted Asparagus 158

Braised Short Ribs 160

Peppercorn-Crusted Beef Short Ribs 162

Soy Ginger Short Ribs with Red Cabbage 164

Cowboy Meatballs. 166

Bison Burgers with Bacon Mayo 167

Pepper Jack Bacon Cheeseburgers. 168

Rib Eye Steak and Pepper Fajitas. 170

Asian Flank Steak Lettuce Wraps. 172

Carne Asada Lettuce Wraps. 174

Prime Rib Roast 176
    Salsa Verde Prime Rib Wraps 177
    Prime Rib Stir-Fry 177
    Prime Rib Cauli-Rice Bowls 178
Rosemary Orange Rib Eye Steaks 179
Beef and Vegetable Kebabs 180
    Beef and Vegetable Kebabs with Olives, Tahini,
    and Cucumber 181
    Chipotle Beef and Vegetable Kebabs with Guacamole 181
Lamb Meatball Wraps with Tzatziki 182

Chapter Nine   DESSERTS 183
Chocolate Chip Cookies 184
Salty Sweet Peanut Butter Cookies 186
All-Butter Shortbread 188
Apple Streusel Bars 190
Raspberry Cream Cheese Bars 192
Slab Pumpkin Pie 194
Slab Cheesecake Four Ways 196
    Cherry Swirl Cheesecake 197
    Peanut Butter Fudge Cheesecake 198
    Chocolate Espresso Swirl Cheesecake 198

Chapter Ten   SAUCES, DIPS, AND OTHER EXTRAS 199
Garlic Herb Compound Butter 200
    Smoky Garlic Butter 201
    Rosemary Orange Butter 201
    Tarragon Butter 202
    Caper Dill Butter 202
Hollandaise Sauce 203
Bacon Mayo 204
Tzatziki 205
Guacamole 206
Salsa Verde 207
Ranch Dip 208
Pesto 209
Marinara Sauce 210

Enchilada Sauce 211

Barbecue Sauce 212

Bacon Mustard Cream Sauce. 213

Teriyaki Sauce 214

Thai Chili Sauce. 215

Spicy Peanut Sauce. 216

Savoy Cabbage and Almond Slaw. 217

Spicy Kale Salad 218

Cauliflower Rice. 220

Mashed Cauliflower 221

CONVERSIONS. 222

ABOUT THE AUTHOR 224

Introduction

When people embark on a low-carb diet for the first time, they often say, "I feel as if I'm saying goodbye to a beloved friend." My goal with this book is to introduce you to a new group of friends—healthy, whole-food, naturally low-carb ingredients and recipes that will love you back. You will lose weight, improve your sleep, and feel better, all while enjoying scrumptious foods.

Chapter 1 provides a brief introduction to the ketogenic diet. It includes the basic carbohydrate guidelines for a keto diet, how to calculate macronutrients, and a list of suitable foods for a ketogenic diet, as well as foods to avoid.

The remainder of the book includes chapters on meals, appetizers, and desserts. Main courses are organized according to the primary source of protein: vegetarian, seafood, poultry, pork, beef, and lamb. The last chapter includes recipes for sauces, dips, and other extras. These things are not prepared on a sheet pan but can be used to accompany sheet-pan meals and also increase the fat content of certain recipes to help you meet your macronutrient goals.

The Ketogenic Diet

What if I told you that you could eat avocados, bacon, butter, and eggs liberally without fear of gaining weight? What if I told you that a diet built around these indulgences could help you prevent—and even reverse—chronic diseases, improve your mood, increase athletic performance, sleep soundly, and effortlessly lose weight without deprivation?

These are the promises of the ketogenic diet. And, boy, are they delicious!

Ketogenic Diet Basics

The ketogenic diet involves shifting your primary fuel source from carbohydrates to fat by limiting the amount of carbs you consume. Ketosis is a normal metabolic process that occurs when glucose is not sufficiently available, and in fact, you are in a light form of ketosis every day between the time you wake up and when you "break your fast" with your first meal. One of the surprising aspects of being in ketosis is that you do not feel hungry. Many people rightly reject the conventional wisdom that eating breakfast is essential for weight loss. Instead, they eat only when they're hungry, allowing the body to draw from its fat stores for energy between meals.

In a low-carb diet—or during periods of fasting or starvation—your blood sugar levels decrease and your liver breaks down fatty acids into ketone bodies, which can be used for energy instead of glucose. In the absence of glucose, ketone bodies can also be used by brain cells. This is important to point out, especially to those who say that our brains need glucose to function. While that is true, they can also function on ketones and may function even better, according to many experts.

For more information on the ketogenic diet, especially as it relates to weight loss, read *The Ketogenic Diet: The Scientifically Proven Approach to Fast, Healthy Weight Loss* by Kristen Mancinelli, MS, RD. There are also infinite resources on the web for maintaining a ketogenic diet.

Macronutrients on a Ketogenic Diet

Most ketogenic diets are not concerned with calories but instead focus on the ratio of macronutrients: fat, protein, and carbohydrate (nevertheless, calorie counts are included with every recipe in this book). The majority of calories on a ketogenic diet should come from fat, about 70 percent. The remaining come from protein, up to 20 to 25 percent, and from carbohydrate, 5 to 7 percent.

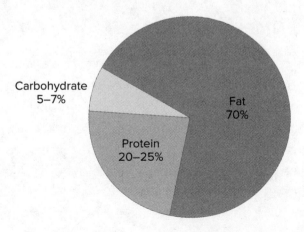

Calculating Carbohydrate

Most experts on the ketogenic diet recommend consuming 20 grams of net carbohydrate or fewer per day, at least initially upon beginning a ketogenic diet. Other experts recommend up to 50 grams of total carbohydrate per day.

Carbohydrates contain 4 calories per gram. The suggested range of 5 to 7 percent carbohydrate on a keto diet would amount to a maximum of 25 to 35 grams of net carbohydrate per day in a 2,000-calorie diet.

There are two methods for calculating carbohydrate in foods. The first is simple and straightforward and involves counting the total amount of carbohydrate in a given food, including fiber. The second method subtracts the grams of fiber from the total amount of carbohydrate, resulting in net carbs.

The total carbohydrate is provided with every recipe in this book along with the grams of fiber, so you can monitor total carbs or net carbs. In this book, all recipes have 15 or fewer grams of net carbs per serving.

How your body responds to dietary carbohydrate is highly individualized. Ultimately, your personal goals and your ketosis monitoring should guide your dietary decisions on how much carbohydrate to eat each day.

Calculating Protein

Achieving and maintaining ketosis requires a low-carbohydrate diet, obviously. However, excess protein can also interfere with ketosis because, to a lesser extent than carbohydrates, protein can increase insulin production.

Protein contains 4 calories per gram. The suggested range of 20 to 25 percent protein on a keto diet would amount to a maximum of 100 to 125 grams of protein per day in a 2,000-calorie diet.

Meat, fish, eggs, nuts, and other foods prevalent on a low-carb diet all contain protein. The trick is balancing the amount of protein with the amount of fat. In this book, I use plenty of free fats such as butter and oil in recipes. However, there is a limit to how much of these fats are palatable or prudent, especially when cooking on a sheet pan. Chapter 10 of this book provides several rich sauces and dips for adding to your sheet-pan meals so you can shift the balance to an even greater percentage of fat.

Calculating Fat

Now comes the fun part! Everyone on a low-fat diet knows just how quickly fat grams and fat calories add up. Even a couple teaspoons of oil for frying your morning egg gives you about 9 grams of fat, not to mention the 5 grams in the egg. At 9 calories per gram, that adds up to a nice 126 calories from fat, or 87 percent of calories from fat.

Remember when you're reading nutrition facts for each recipe that even though the grams of protein and fat may be about equal, fat has more than double the calories per gram. So, 25 grams of protein equal 100 calories, whereas 25 grams of fat equal 225 calories.

Ketogenic Diet Foods

The ketogenic diet includes a surprisingly wide array of fresh vegetables, meat, seafood, nuts, and dairy products. It can even include a limited amount of berries and other low-sugar fruits. Here are the basic foods included on a ketogenic diet.

VEGETABLES AND FRUIT

- Artichoke
- Arugula
- Asparagus
- Avocado
- Berries
- Bok choy

- Broccoli
- Brussels sprouts
- Cabbage
- Cauliflower
- Celery
- Collard greens
- Cucumber
- Endive
- Fennel
- Garlic
- Ginger
- Herbs
- Kale
- Leeks
- Lettuce
- Mushrooms
- Onions
- Peppers
- Radish
- Spinach
- Tomato
- Watercress
- Zucchini

MEAT

- Beef (steaks, ribs, ground, etc.)
- Bison
- Chicken (breasts, thighs, legs, liver, sausage, etc.)
- Lamb
- Pork (bacon, sausage, ground, pork belly, ribs, etc.)

SEAFOOD

- Clams
- Halibut
- Mussels
- Oysters
- Salmon
- Scallops
- Shrimp

NUTS AND SEEDS

- Almonds
- Cashews
- Macadamia nuts
- Pecans
- Pistachios
- Sesame seeds
- Walnuts

DAIRY AND EGGS

- Butter
- Cheese (Brie, Parmesan, cheddar, fontina, mozzarella, etc.)
- Cottage cheese
- Cream
- Eggs
- Full-fat cream cheese
- Full-fat sour cream
- Full-fat yogurt
- Whole milk

FATS

- Butter
- Coconut oil
- Ghee
- Lard
- Mayonnaise
- Olive oil
- Vegetable oil

What Not to Eat

Some of these probably go without saying, but here are some of the foods that don't fit well within the ketogenic diet. That's not to say that you cannot ever have them, but they contain so many carbohydrates that even in small doses they will stall or even prevent ketosis:

- Beans
- Bread
- Chickpeas
- Fruit juice
- High-fructose corn syrup
- Lentils
- Pasta
- Pastries
- Potatoes
- Quinoa
- Refined sugar
- Rice
- Soda
- Sweet potatoes
- Wheat
- Most processed foods
- Most high-sugar fruits (except berries)
- Other starchy vegetables such as corn, parsnips, and peas

Stocking Your Pantry

Stocking your pantry for ketogenic cooking isn't very different from preparing for other methods of cooking. The ingredients below appear often in the recipes in this book. Having them in your pantry or refrigerator will make low-carb cooking even easier.

Oils and vinegars: When a neutral flavor is desired, I usually cook with canola oil. Coconut oil is good in low-carb desserts or for providing a coconut flavor. I use olive oil when its flavor is desirable in cooking, though I reserve extra-virgin olive oil for finishing a dish or using in salad dressings. Vinegars such as red wine vinegar, balsamic vinegar, and apple cider vinegar add brightness to food and are used throughout this cookbook.

Dairy: Butter can be used as a cooking fat, to infuse food with flavor, and for finishing sauces. I do not specify unsalted or salted butter in these recipes; use whatever you have on hand. Also, stock your refrigerator with heavy cream, full-fat sour cream, and Parmesan cheese. When it is used for breading, canned Parmesan works better than the finer block-variety, but both are nice to have on hand.

Nuts: Store fresh almonds, cashews, macadamia nuts, and pecans in the pantry. Either raw or toasted is okay. Pistachios and walnuts are nice as well, but not essential to the recipes in this book.

Condiments: Stock Dijon mustard and full-fat real mayonnaise in your pantry or, if opened, in your refrigerator. Soy sauce is also used in these recipes, so choose a gluten-free soy sauce if you need to eat a gluten-free diet.

Baking: I use liquid stevia in the recipes in this book. A little goes a long way, so a 1-ounce bottle should be enough to get you started. Shredded coconut can be used in baking and for breading foods. Coconut milk is a nice dairy-free, high-fat option for baking and making curries or sauces. Almond flour and coconut flour are essential for low-carb baking.

Miscellaneous: Low-carb wraps are nice to have on hand to transform leftovers into a nice lunch. They are used occasionally in the recipes in this book. Look for a variety with about 70 calories and 5 grams of carbs per serving.

Equipment

For the recipes in this book, the primary piece of equipment you'll need is a rimmed sheet pan about 12 by 16 inches, referred to as a half sheet pan in the restaurant industry. I also often call for parchment paper for lining the pan. This allows for easy removal of food from the pan and makes cleanup a breeze.

You will also need a few mixing bowls, a cutting board, and of course, a chef's knife for chopping.

Recipe Labels

Recipes in this book that are fewer than 500 calories per serving contain the label "low calorie." I have also included the labels gluten free, dairy free, and vegetarian for navigating dietary restrictions.

CHAPTER TWO

Breakfast

The standard American breakfast is typically loaded with carbs in the form of sugary breakfast cereals and pastries, high-glycemic bagels and toast, and pancakes and waffles drowning in syrup. Wash it all down with sugared coffee or sweetened juice, and it's a blood sugar nightmare! It's time to take breakfast in a new direction. These ketogenic breakfasts will satisfy your hunger and keep your blood sugar stable until lunchtime.

CINNAMON NUT GRANOLA

When I transitioned to a grain-free diet several years ago, I especially missed my favorite breakfast—crunchy granola and fruit over tangy, cool yogurt. This version satisfies my cravings and is delicious with a small handful of low-sugar fruit, such as raspberries or blackberries. Use coconut oil instead of butter for a dairy-free option.

YIELD: 12 (½-cup) servings   PREP TIME: 5 minutes
COOK TIME: 25 minutes

2 cups pecans

2 cups almonds

2 cups walnuts

1 egg white, whisked

2 teaspoons ground cinnamon

½ cup coconut oil or melted butter

1 teaspoon vanilla extract

1 teaspoon liquid stevia

⅛ teaspoon sea salt

1. Preheat the oven to 325°F.

2. Place the pecans, almonds, and walnuts in a food processor and pulse until the mixture is coarsely ground, about the size of old-fashioned rolled oats.

3. In a medium bowl, combine the egg white, cinnamon, coconut oil or butter, vanilla, stevia, and sea salt. Whisk until thoroughly mixed.

4. Pour the liquid ingredients into the food processor and pulse a few times, just until all ingredients are integrated.

5. Pour the mixture onto a sheet pan and flatten gently with a metal spatula.

6. Bake for 10 minutes. Stir the mixture and flatten again with the spatula. Return the pan to the oven and bake for 10 minutes.

7. Flip the mixture, trying to keep the pieces intact as if flipping pancakes. Return to the oven and bake for another 5 minutes.

8. Remove the pan from the oven. Allow the granola to cool completely on the pan, then transfer to an airtight container and store.

GLUTEN FREE · VEGETARIAN · DAIRY FREE · LOW CALORIE

Nutrition Facts (amount per serving)	
Calories	462
Fat	46 g
Protein	10 g
Carbohydrate	10 g
Fiber	6 g

PUMPKIN SPICE GRANOLA

Pumpkin pie spice complements so many foods, with or without the addition of pumpkin puree. This recipe uses a scant half-cup of pumpkin to keep carbs down, though it provides a generous dose of the spice blend. If you don't have pumpkin pie spice on hand, make your own using the recipe in the tip. Use coconut oil instead of butter for a dairy-free option.

YIELD: 12 (½-cup) servings   PREP TIME: 5 minutes
COOK TIME: 25 minutes

3 cups pecans

2 cups almonds

1 cup pumpkin seeds

½ cup pumpkin puree

1 tablespoon pumpkin pie spice

1 egg white, whisked

¼ cup coconut oil or melted butter

1 teaspoon vanilla extract

1 teaspoon liquid stevia

⅛ teaspoon sea salt

1. Preheat the oven to 325°F.

2. Place the pecans and almonds in a food processor and pulse until the mixture is coarsely ground, about the size of old-fashioned rolled oats. Add the pumpkin seeds to the food processor.

3. In a medium bowl, combine the pumpkin puree, pumpkin pie spice, egg white, coconut oil or butter, vanilla, stevia, and sea salt. Whisk until thoroughly mixed.

4. Pour the liquid ingredients into the food processor and pulse a few times, just until all ingredients are integrated.

5. Pour the mixture onto a sheet pan and flatten gently with a metal spatula.

6. Bake for 10 minutes. Stir the mixture and flatten again with the spatula. Return the pan to the oven and bake for 10 minutes.

7. Flip the mixture, trying to keep the pieces intact as if flipping pancakes. Return to the oven and bake for another 5 minutes.

8. Remove the pan from the oven. Allow the granola to cool completely on the pan, then transfer to an airtight container and store.

GLUTEN FREE · VEGETARIAN · DAIRY FREE · LOW CALORIE

Nutrition Facts	
(amount per serving)	
Calories	425
Fat	41 g
Protein	12 g
Carbohydrate	10 g
Fiber	6 g

INGREDIENT TIP: To make your own pumpkin pie spice blend, combine 1 tablespoon ground cinnamon, 2 teaspoons ground ginger, 1 teaspoon ground nutmeg, ½ teaspoon ground allspice, and ½ teaspoon ground cloves. Store in a covered container.

TROPICAL COCONUT GRANOLA

Macadamia nuts and shredded coconut bring tropical flavors to this nut granola. If you can find pineapple extract, it adds another layer of flavor, but the granola is delicious without it.

YIELD: 12 (½-cup) servings   PREP TIME: 5 minutes
COOK TIME: 25 minutes

2 cups macadamia nuts

2 cups almonds

2 cups shredded
unsweetened coconut

1 egg white, whisked

½ cup coconut oil

1 teaspoon vanilla extract

¼ teaspoon pineapple
extract (optional)

1 teaspoon liquid stevia

⅛ teaspoon sea salt

1. Preheat the oven to 325°F.

2. Place the macadamia nuts and almonds in a food processor and pulse until the mixture is coarsely ground, about the size of old-fashioned rolled oats. Add the coconut to the food processor.

3. In a medium bowl, combine the egg white, coconut oil, vanilla, pineapple extract (if using), stevia, and sea salt. Whisk until thoroughly mixed.

4. Pour the liquid ingredients into the food processor and pulse a few times, just until all ingredients are integrated.

5. Pour the mixture onto a sheet pan and flatten gently with a metal spatula.

6. Bake for 10 minutes. Stir the mixture and flatten again with the spatula. Return the pan to the oven and bake for 10 minutes.

7. Flip the mixture, trying to keep the pieces intact as if flipping pancakes. Return to the oven and bake for another 5 minutes.

SHEET PAN KETOGENIC

8. Remove the pan from the oven. Allow the granola to cool completely on the pan, then transfer to an airtight container and store.

GLUTEN FREE • VEGETARIAN • DAIRY FREE • LOW CALORIE

Nutrition Facts	
(amount per serving)	
Calories	465
Fat	47 g
Protein	8 g
Carbohydrate	12 g
Fiber	7 g

BASIC CLOUD BREAD

Cloud bread is the keto dieter's best friend, making it easy to put sandwiches, burgers, and pizzas back on the menu. The bread is naturally grain- and nut-free, and gets its volume from whipped egg whites. As its name suggests, it is light and airy in texture. Depending on how sweet you want the bread, add more or less stevia. But remember, a little goes a long way!

YIELD: 9 servings   PREP TIME: 10 minutes   COOK TIME: 30 minutes

3 eggs, divided

¼ teaspoon cream of tartar

sea salt

3 tablespoons cream cheese

1 or 2 drops liquid stevia

1. Preheat the oven to 300°F. Line a sheet pan with parchment paper.

2. In a medium bowl, whip the egg whites, cream of tartar, and a pinch of sea salt until stiff peaks form, about 3 minutes.

3. In a large bowl, beat the egg yolks, cream cheese, and liquid stevia until smooth.

4. Transfer about one-third of the egg whites into the egg yolk mixture to lighten it. Stir until thoroughly integrated.

5. Fold in the remaining egg whites and stir just until blended, trying not to deflate the egg whites.

6. Place the mixture onto the sheet pan in 9 scoops. Use the back of a spoon to spread them out into circles about 3 to 4 inches in diameter.

7. Bake for 30 minutes, until the breads are set and the tops are gently browned.

GLUTEN FREE · VEGETARIAN · LOW CALORIE

Nutrition Facts	
(amount per serving)	
Calories	41
Fat	3 g
Protein	3 g
Carbohydrate	0 g
Fiber	0 g

CLOUD BREAD AVOCADO TOAST

1. Prepare the Basic Cloud Bread.

2. Place a piece of the bread in a toaster and toast for 45 to 60 seconds, being careful not to burn.

3. Top with 1 tablespoon softened cream cheese and ½ avocado, thinly sliced. Season with salt and pepper.

GLUTEN FREE • VEGETARIAN • LOW CALORIE

Nutrition Facts	
(amount per serving)	
Calories	221
Fat	18 g
Protein	3 g
Carbohydrate	5 g
Fiber	3.5 g

CLOUD BREAD BLT

1. Prepare the Basic Cloud Bread.

2. Coat one side of one piece of cloud bread with 1 tablespoon mayonnaise.

3. Top with 2 slices cooked bacon, 2 thin slices tomato, and 2 lettuce leaves.

4. Coat one side of another piece of cloud bread with 1 tablespoon mayonnaise and place it on top of the lettuce to form a sandwich.

GLUTEN FREE • LOW CALORIE

Nutrition Facts	
(amount per serving)	
Calories	423
Fat	40 g
Protein	17 g
Carbohydrate	2.4 g
Fiber	0.8 g

CLOUD BREAD EGGS BENEDICT

1. Prepare the Basic Cloud Bread.

2. Set one piece on a plate.

3. Top with 1 fried egg and 2 tablespoons of Hollandaise Sauce (page 203). Season with salt and pepper.

GLUTEN FREE ▪ VEGETARIAN ▪ LOW CALORIE

Nutrition Facts	
(amount per serving)	
Calories	363
Fat	35 g
Protein	11 g
Carbohydrate	1 g
Fiber	0 g

APPLE SAGE PORK SAUSAGE

Fresh sage and minced apple bring complexity and sweetness to these easy breakfast sausages.

YIELD: 4 servings   PREP TIME: 5 minutes   COOK TIME: 18 to 20 minutes

1 pound ground pork

1 tablespoon minced fresh sage

1 tablespoon minced shallot

1 small tart apple, peeled, cored, and finely grated

¾ teaspoon sea salt

¼ teaspoon freshly ground pepper

1. Preheat the oven to 375°F. Line a sheet pan with parchment paper.

2. Combine the pork, sage, shallot, apple, sea salt, and pepper in a small bowl. Use your hands to thoroughly mix.

3. Form the mixture into 8 small patties and place them on a sheet pan. Bake for 18 to 20 minutes or until cooked to an internal temperature of 145°F.

GLUTEN FREE · DAIRY FREE · LOW CALORIE

Nutrition Facts	
(amount per serving)	
Calories	349
Fat	24 g
Protein	29 g
Carbohydrate	3 g
Fiber	1 g

SAVORY BREAKFAST SAUSAGE

This homemade pork sausage is big on flavor and light on carbs. It is delicious crumbled into a breakfast scramble or wrapped in a low-carb wrap.

YIELD: 4 servings   PREP TIME: 5 minutes   COOK TIME: 18 to 20 minutes

1 pound ground pork

1 teaspoon minced fresh thyme

1 teaspoon minced fresh rosemary

1 tablespoon minced fresh parsley

1 teaspoon minced garlic

pinch red chile flakes

¾ teaspoon sea salt

¼ teaspoon freshly ground pepper

1. Preheat the oven to 375°F. Line a sheet pan with parchment paper.

2. Combine the pork, thyme, rosemary, parsley, garlic, red chile flakes, sea salt, and pepper in a small bowl. Use your hands to thoroughly mix.

3. Form the mixture into 8 small patties and place them on a sheet pan. Bake for 18 to 20 minutes or until cooked to an internal temperature of 145°F.

GLUTEN FREE ▪ DAIRY FREE ▪ LOW CALORIE

Nutrition Facts	
(amount per serving)	
Calories	349
Fat	24 g
Protein	29 g
Carbohydrate	3 g
Fiber	1 g

GREEN SHAKSHUKA WITH HERBS AND ZA'ATAR

This flavorful breakfast dish combines bell peppers, onions, and fresh herbs. It is topped with barely cooked eggs and is popular throughout the Mediterranean. Serve with a low-carb bread to sop up all of the juices. Za'atar is a Middle Eastern spice that combines dried herbs, sesame seeds, and sumac. If you can't find it, use a pinch of red chile flakes, sesame seeds, and ground oregano.

YIELD: 4 servings   PREP TIME: 10 minutes   COOK TIME: 15 to 25 minutes

4 green bell peppers, sliced in long strips

2 yellow onions, sliced in half circles

2 tablespoons olive oil

sea salt

freshly ground pepper

8 eggs

½ cup roughly chopped fresh cilantro

½ cup roughly chopped fresh parsley

2 teaspoons za'atar

1. Preheat the oven to 375°F.

2. Combine the peppers and onions on a sheet pan. Drizzle with olive oil and toss to coat thoroughly. Season with salt and pepper.

3. Roast uncovered for 15 to 20 minutes, stirring once or twice.

4. Remove the pan from the oven and push the vegetables to the side to make 8 small "wells." Crack the eggs into each space and return to the oven to cook for another 5 minutes or until the egg whites are set. Shower with the fresh cilantro and parsley and sprinkle with the za'atar.

GLUTEN FREE · VEGETARIAN · DAIRY FREE · LOW CALORIE

Nutrition Facts	
(amount per serving)	
Calories	245
Fat	17 g
Protein	14 g
Carbohydrate	11 g
Fiber	1 g

TRADITIONAL SHAKSHUKA

Use yellow and red bell peppers instead of green, and add 1 pint grape tomatoes. Skip the za'atar and use ½ teaspoon ground cumin and ½ teaspoon smoked paprika.

GLUTEN FREE · VEGETARIAN · DAIRY FREE · LOW CALORIE

Nutrition Facts	
(amount per serving)	
Calories	262
Fat	17 g
Protein	14 g
Carbohydrate	6 g
Fiber	1.6 g

MUSHROOM, SUN-DRIED TOMATO, AND HERB FRITTATA

Savory mushrooms, sweet sun-dried tomatoes, and grassy herbs permeate this simple vegetarian breakfast.

YIELD: 4 servings   PREP TIME: 10 minutes   COOK TIME: 20 to 22 minutes

16 ounces cremini mushrooms, quartered

1 tablespoon olive oil

¼ cup minced sun-dried tomatoes

2 tablespoons minced fresh parsley

2 scallions, sliced thinly on a bias

1 dozen eggs

sea salt

freshly ground pepper

1. Preheat the oven to 375°F.

2. Toss the mushrooms with the olive oil on the sheet pan. Sprinkle with the sun-dried tomatoes, parsley, and scallions. Season with salt and pepper. Roast uncovered for 10 minutes.

3. Combine the eggs in a large pitcher and whisk until nearly combined. Season with salt.

4. Pour the eggs into the sheet pan and return to the oven for 10 to 12 minutes or until the eggs are nearly set. Allow to rest for 5 minutes before cutting and serving.

GLUTEN FREE • VEGETARIAN • DAIRY FREE • LOW CALORIE

Nutrition Facts	
(amount per serving)	
Calories	360
Fat	25 g
Protein	27 g
Carbohydrate	9 g
Fiber	2.2 g

SAUSAGE, ROSEMARY, AND ROASTED ONION FRITTATA

Savory pork sausage, delicate zucchini, and fragrant rosemary make this frittata a decadent, but still decidedly low-carb, breakfast option. It's perfect for a lazy weekend brunch, served with nothing more than a strong cup of coffee.

YIELD: 4 servings   PREP TIME: 10 minutes   COOK TIME: 25 to 27 minutes

16 ounces pork sausage, cut into 1-inch pieces

1 red onion, halved and thinly sliced

2 medium zucchini, cut into 1-inch pieces

1 tablespoon olive oil

1 tablespoon minced fresh rosemary

1 dozen eggs

sea salt

freshly ground pepper

1. Preheat the oven to 375°F.

2. Spread the pork, onion, and zucchini onto a sheet pan. Drizzle with the olive oil, tossing gently to coat. Season with the rosemary, salt, and pepper. Roast uncovered for 15 minutes or until the sausage is cooked through.

3. Combine the eggs in a large pitcher and whisk until nearly combined. Season with salt.

4. Pour the eggs into the sheet pan and return to the oven for 10 to 12 minutes or until the eggs are nearly set. Allow to rest for 5 minutes before cutting and serving.

GLUTEN FREE · DAIRY FREE

Nutrition Facts	
(amount per serving)	
Calories	558
Fat	41 g
Protein	36 g
Carbohydrate	8 g
Fiber	1.9 g

BAKED EGGS IN AVOCADO

*Using slightly under-ripe avocados is your best bet for these flavor-
ful baked avocados. Start with the basic version of eggs baked in
avocado and then take this dish in three different directions—spicy
harissa, salmon and dill, or classic bacon and cheese.*

YIELD: 4 servings   PREP TIME: 5 minutes   COOK TIME: 15 minutes

2 large avocados, halved
vertically, pits removed

4 medium eggs

sea salt

freshly ground pepper

1. Preheat the oven to 425°F.

2. Place the avocado halves cut-side up on a sheet pan. If the inden-
tation from the pit is small, make it slightly larger by scooping out
some of the avocado flesh with a spoon.

3. Crack an egg into each avocado half. Season with salt and pepper.

4. Carefully transfer the pan to the oven. Bake for 15 minutes or until
the egg whites are set.

GLUTEN FREE · VEGETARIAN · DAIRY FREE · LOW CALORIE

Nutrition Facts	
(amount per serving)	
Calories	205
Fat	17 g
Protein	8 g
Carbohydrate	7 g
Fiber	5.4 g

SPICY HARISSA BAKED EGGS IN AVOCADO

Make the basic recipe for Baked Eggs in Avocado. Before adding the
egg, spoon 1 tablespoon of harissa into each avocado.

GLUTEN FREE · VEGETARIAN · DAIRY FREE · LOW CALORIE

Nutrition Facts	
(amount per serving)	
Calories	209
Fat	17 g
Protein	8 g
Carbohydrate	8 g
Fiber	5.4 g

SALMON AND DILL BAKED EGGS IN AVOCADO

Prepare and cook the basic recipe for Baked Eggs in Avocado and top each egg with a thin slice of smoked salmon and a sprig of fresh dill.

GLUTEN FREE ▪ DAIRY FREE ▪ LOW CALORIE

Nutrition Facts	
(amount per serving)	
Calories	222
Fat	18 g
Protein	11 g
Carbohydrate	7 g
Fiber	5.4 g

BACON AND CHEESE BAKED EGGS IN AVOCADO

Make the basic recipe for Baked Eggs in Avocado. Before baking, sprinkle each egg with 1 tablespoon cheddar cheese. After baking, top each avocado half with 1 tablespoon sour cream and 1 tablespoon bacon bits.

GLUTEN FREE ▪ LOW CALORIE

Nutrition Facts	
(amount per serving)	
Calories	313
Fat	26 g
Protein	15 g
Carbohydrate	8 g
Fiber	5.4 g

CHAPTER THREE

Snacks and Appetizers

One of the benefits of a ketogenic diet is that you rarely feel hungry between meals. Nevertheless, sometimes it's nice to have something to nibble on after an intense workout or while you prepare a more sizeable meal. Here are some of my favorite sides, snacks, and appetizers. Some can be made into complete meals by adding nothing more than a piece of meat or fish to the pan.

ALMOND PARMESAN CRISPS

Serve these crisps as part of a cheese and meat platter. The tarragon can be replaced with thyme, basil, or rosemary, but it's worth the effort to find fresh tarragon, as it works so well with the Parmesan.

YIELD: 8 servings   PREP TIME: 5 minutes   COOK TIME: 10 to 12 minutes

1½ cups blanched almond flour

1 cup grated Parmesan cheese

1 tablespoon minced fresh tarragon (optional)

¼ teaspoon sea salt

2 tablespoons olive oil

1 to 2 tablespoons ice water

1. Preheat the oven to 325°F. Cut two pieces of parchment paper the same size as your sheet pan.

2. Combine the almond flour, Parmesan, tarragon, and sea salt in a large bowl. Stir in the olive oil. Add the ice water a teaspoon at a time, stirring until the mixture comes together as a ball. It should be fairly dry.

3. Place the dough onto one sheet of parchment paper and place the second sheet of parchment over the top. Use a rolling pin to roll the dough as thinly as possible. Carefully peel away the top sheet of parchment.

4. Use a chef's knife to cut the dough into 32 crackers. Slide the parchment onto a sheet pan.

5. Bake for 10 minutes, or until beginning to turn golden. Do not overbake.

GLUTEN FREE · VEGETARIAN · LOW CALORIE

Nutrition Facts	
(amount per serving)	
Calories	209
Fat	18 g
Protein	10 g
Carbohydrate	5 g
Fiber	2.3 g

VEGAN ROSEMARY HAZELNUT CRISPS

Prepare the Almond Parmesan Crisps but use 2 cups hazelnut flour and 1 teaspoon minced rosemary in place of the almond flour, tarragon, and Parmesan cheese.

GLUTEN FREE • VEGETARIAN • DAIRY FREE • LOW CALORIE

Nutrition Facts	
(amount per serving)	
Calories	210
Fat	20 g
Protein	4 g
Carbohydrate	5 g
Fiber	3 g

SPICED MIXED NUTS

As much as I love plain raw nuts, roasting them in a simple spicy and sweet sauce makes them absolutely addicting. It is the perfect low-carb party appetizer or on-the-go snack.

YIELD: 12 (¼-cup) servings   PREP TIME: 5 minutes
COOK TIME: 10 to 12 minutes

1 cup pecans

1 cup cashews

1 cup almonds

⅓ cup coconut oil

¼ teaspoon liquid stevia

2 tablespoons hot sauce, such as Cholula

1 teaspoon sea salt

1. Preheat the oven to 350°F. Line a sheet pan with parchment paper.

2. Combine the nuts in a large bowl. In a medium bowl, whisk together the oil, stevia, hot sauce, and sea salt. Pour over the nuts and toss to coat thoroughly.

3. Spread the mixture out over the sheet pan and bake for 10 to 12 minutes, stirring once. Allow to cool thoroughly before enjoying.

GLUTEN FREE ▪ VEGETARIAN ▪ DAIRY FREE ▪ LOW CALORIE

Nutrition Facts	
(amount per serving)	
Calories	179
Fat	18 g
Protein	3 g
Carbohydrate	5 g
Fiber	1.2 g

ZUCCHINI ONION LATKES

Typically, latkes are made with potatoes. This version opts for onions and zucchini and tops them with full-fat sour cream for a delicious low-carb snack.

YIELD: 4 servings   PREP TIME: 5 minutes   COOK TIME: 30 minutes

2 zucchini, grated

1 yellow onion, grated

1 egg, whisked

1 tablespoon coconut flour

¼ teaspoon baking powder

sea salt

freshly ground pepper

½ cup full-fat sour cream

1. Preheat the oven to 400°F. Line a sheet pan with parchment paper.

2. Squeeze the moisture out of the zucchini and onion with your hands over a colander in the sink.

3. In a medium bowl, combine the egg, coconut flour, and baking powder. Season with salt and pepper. Fold in the grated zucchini and onion.

4. Form the mixture into 8 small patties and set them on the sheet pan.

5. Bake for 20 minutes. Carefully flip the patties and bake for another 10 minutes until browned and crisp.

6. Serve with sour cream.

GLUTEN FREE · VEGETARIAN · LOW CALORIE

Nutrition Facts	
(amount per serving)	
Calories	112
Fat	8 g
Protein	4 g
Carbohydrate	8 g
Fiber	2.6 g

GARLIC AND LEMON ROASTED CAULIFLOWER

I can't get enough of this flavorful plant-based appetizer. It is one of my standbys for tapas night.

YIELD: 4 servings   PREP TIME: 10 minutes   COOK TIME: 30 minutes

1 head cauliflower, broken or cut into small florets

2 cloves garlic, finely minced

zest and juice of 1 lemon

¼ cup olive oil

¼ cup roughly chopped fresh parsley

sea salt

freshly ground pepper

1. Preheat the oven to 375°F.

2. In a large bowl, combine the cauliflower with the garlic, lemon zest, and olive oil. Spread out over the sheet pan. Season generously with salt and pepper.

3. Roast for 30 minutes uncovered or until the cauliflower browns on the bottom and shrivels slightly.

4. Shower the roasted cauliflower with parsley and lemon juice. Serve warm.

GLUTEN FREE • VEGETARIAN • DAIRY FREE • LOW CALORIE

Nutrition Facts	
(amount per serving)	
Calories	163
Fat	14 g
Protein	3 g
Carbohydrate	9 g
Fiber	3.8 g

ROASTED CAULIFLOWER WITH MINT AND PINE NUTS

Prepare the Garlic and Lemon Roasted Cauliflower but use mint instead of fresh parsley and shower with 2 tablespoons of crushed toasted pine nuts.

GLUTEN FREE · VEGETARIAN · DAIRY FREE · LOW CALORIE

Nutrition Facts	
(amount per serving)	
Calories	187
Fat	20 g
Protein	10 g
Carbohydrate	6 g
Fiber	2.7 g

BROILED ROMAINE HEARTS WITH ROASTED PEPPERS

Give this salad standby a lively upgrade! When you halve and broil romaine, the inner leaves char to become gently wilted and crispy along the edges. Topped with roasted red peppers and Kalamata olives, romaine is fresh and fun.

YIELD: 8 servings   PREP TIME: 10 minutes   COOK TIME: 2 minutes

2 romaine lettuce hearts

2 tablespoons olive oil, divided

1 shallot or small red onion, thinly sliced

1 teaspoon minced fresh thyme

juice of 1 lemon

2 roasted red peppers, thinly sliced

¼ cup pitted Kalamata olives

sea salt

freshly ground pepper

1. Place an oven rack on the top level and preheat the broiler to high.

2. Slice the romaine hearts lengthwise and brush with 1 tablespoon of the olive oil. Set them on the sheet pan. Season with salt and pepper. Broil for 1 to 2 minutes or until the top of the lettuce is lightly charred.

3. In a small bowl, make the dressing by combining the remaining olive oil, shallot or red onion, thyme, and lemon juice. Season with salt and pepper.

4. To serve, top each romaine heart with the sliced red peppers and olives, and drizzle with the dressing.

GLUTEN FREE · VEGETARIAN · DAIRY FREE · LOW CALORIE

Nutrition Facts	
(amount per serving)	
Calories	131
Fat	11 g
Protein	2 g
Carbohydrate	8 g
Fiber	2.4 g

SMOKY SWEET ROASTED CABBAGE

I love preparing this recipe on the grill, but when the weather is cool and it gets dark before the dinner hour, I take things inside. Oven roasting produces a similar effect and there's no danger of food falling through the grate.

YIELD: 4 servings   PREP TIME: 5 minutes   COOK TIME: 45 minutes

1 small red cabbage	1 teaspoon smoked paprika
¼ cup balsamic vinegar	2 tablespoons canola oil
2 teaspoons Dijon mustard	sea salt
1 teaspoon ground cumin	freshly ground pepper

1. Preheat the oven to 400°F. Line a sheet pan with parchment paper.

2. Slice the cabbage into 16 wedges, being sure to allow each one to retain a small portion of the core. This will help them hold together.

3. Whisk the balsamic, Dijon, cumin, smoked paprika, and oil together in a small bowl. Season with salt and pepper.

4. Lay the cabbage slices on the parchment paper. Drizzle with the balsamic vinaigrette.

5. Bake for 25 minutes before turning the cabbage over. Bake for another 20 minutes until the cabbage is tender and gently browned.

GLUTEN FREE ▪ VEGAN ▪ DAIRY FREE ▪ LOW CALORIE

Nutrition Facts	
(amount per serving)	
Calories	111
Fat	7 g
Protein	2 g
Carbohydrate	10 g
Fiber	4 g

CHORIZO-STUFFED MUSHROOMS

These roasted mushrooms are stuffed with spicy Spanish chorizo, tangy Manchego cheese, and garlic and herbs. Chorizo is available raw in bulk or in a cured, ready-to-eat version that can be sliced and eaten as a tapa or added to recipes. Manchego cheese is a Spanish sheep's milk cheese that holds its shape when baked, instead of oozing all over the place.

YIELD: 4 servings   PREP TIME: 5 minutes   COOK TIME: 25 minutes

4 ounces cured Spanish chorizo, finely diced

1 pound cremini mushrooms, about 24 caps

2 cloves garlic, minced

1 shallot, minced

2 tablespoons minced fresh parsley

1 ounce Manchego cheese, grated

sea salt

freshly ground pepper

1. Preheat the oven to 350°F. Line a sheet pan with parchment paper.

2. Place the chorizo in a small bowl.

3. Remove the stems from the mushrooms and mince them. Add them to the bowl along with the garlic, shallot, parsley, and Manchego. Season with salt and pepper.

4. Divide the mixture between the mushroom caps and place them on a sheet pan.

5. Bake for 25 minutes or until the mushrooms are soft and the filling is bubbling and browned.

GLUTEN FREE • LOW CALORIE

Nutrition Facts	
(amount per serving)	
Calories	182
Fat	13 g
Protein	12 g
Carbohydrate	6 g
Fiber	1.4 g

CHEESY ARTICHOKE-STUFFED MUSHROOMS

Prepare the recipe for Chorizo-Stuffed Mushrooms, but replace the chorizo with ½ cup roughly chopped artichoke hearts and an additional 1 ounce of Manchego cheese.

GLUTEN FREE · VEGETARIAN · LOW CALORIE

Nutrition Facts	
(amount per serving)	
Calories	139
Fat	8 g
Protein	8 g
Carbohydrate	12 g
Fiber	1.6 g

ASPARAGUS WITH HAZELNUT ROMESCO

The flavors in this pungent chile and tomato sauce will make you want to keep the entire appetizer to yourself.

YIELD: 4 servings   PREP TIME: 10 minutes   COOK TIME: 35 to 38 minutes

1 red bell pepper, cored and halved lengthwise

1 Fresno chile, cored and halved lengthwise

6 cloves garlic, unpeeled

1 pint grape tomatoes, divided

5 tablespoons olive oil, divided

2 teaspoons red wine vinegar

1 bunch asparagus, about 20 large spears

4 tablespoons roughly chopped toasted hazelnuts, divided

½ teaspoon smoked paprika

sea salt

freshly ground pepper

1. Preheat the oven to 400°F. Line a sheet pan with parchment paper.

2. Place the bell pepper, Fresno chile, garlic cloves, and the grape tomatoes on one side of the pan, reserving about 4 tomatoes for a garnish. Drizzle with 2 tablespoons of the olive oil and season with salt and pepper. Roast for 20 minutes.

3. Remove the Fresno chile and garlic from the pan and turn the red pepper over.

4. Peel the garlic cloves and place them into a blender with the chile, 2 tablespoons of olive oil, and the red wine vinegar.

5. Add the asparagus to the other side of the sheet pan with the red pepper and toss with 1 tablespoon of olive oil. Season with salt and pepper. Return the pan to the oven and roast for another 15 to 18 minutes, until the asparagus are tender and beginning to brown.

6. Peel the red pepper. Add the pepper and tomatoes to the blender with the chile and garlic. Add 3 tablespoons of the hazelnuts and the smoked paprika to the blender and puree until smooth, adding more olive oil if needed to get things going.

7. To serve, pour the sauce over the roasted asparagus and garnish with the remaining tomatoes and hazelnuts.

GLUTEN FREE ▪ VEGETARIAN ▪ DAIRY FREE ▪ LOW CALORIE

Nutrition Facts	
(amount per serving)	
Calories	263
Fat	22 g
Protein	4 g
Carbohydrate	16 g
Fiber	3.3 g

ROASTED ASPARAGUS WITH POACHED EGG

Prepare the recipe for Asparagus with Hazelnut Romesco. Serve topped with 2 poached or fried eggs per serving to make a filling lunch or light dinner.

GLUTEN FREE ▪ VEGETARIAN ▪ DAIRY FREE ▪ LOW CALORIE

Nutrition Facts	
(amount per serving)	
Calories	383
Fat	32 g
Protein	16 g
Carbohydrate	16 g
Fiber	3.3 g

PROSCIUTTO-WRAPPED ASPARAGUS

If asparagus isn't your thing, wrap it in prosciutto and you may just change your mind. The vegetable is naturally low-carb and a good source of fiber, making it a good option on a ketogenic diet. Choose medium asparagus spears that are neither very thin nor thick and woody. This makes a festive party appetizer or scrumptious side dish.

YIELD: 4 servings   PREP TIME: 5 minutes   COOK TIME: 12 to 15 minutes

1 tablespoon olive oil

1 bunch asparagus, about 20 large spears

10 slices prosciutto

1. Preheat the oven to 425°F. Coat the sheet pan with the olive oil.

2. Trim the asparagus spears by snapping off the woody ends at the point at which they break.

3. Slice each of the prosciutto slices in half lengthwise.

4. Wrap each asparagus spear in a slice of prosciutto, beginning about 1 inch below the tip of the asparagus. Place each spear on the sheet pan.

5. Bake for 12 to 15 minutes until the asparagus is barely tender and the prosciutto is crisp.

GLUTEN FREE ▪ DAIRY FREE ▪ LOW CALORIE

Nutrition Facts	
(amount per serving)	
Calories	123
Fat	9 g
Protein	8 g
Carbohydrate	6 g
Fiber	2 g

AVOCADO BACON FRIES

Try these quick and easy oven fries made with just two ingredients. They're crisp on the outside with a creamy filling. And you thought regular French fries were decadent! Make sure to choose thin-cut bacon so that it cooks quickly in the oven. Serve with Ranch Dip (page 208).

YIELD: 4 servings   PREP TIME: 5 minutes   COOK TIME: 10 minutes

8 slices thin-cut bacon, about 6 ounces

2 avocados, peeled and cut
into 8 wedges each

1. Preheat the oven to 400°F. Line a sheet pan with parchment paper.

2. Cut each slice of bacon in half so that you have a total of 16 slices.

3. Wrap each avocado spear with a slice of bacon and place on the sheet pan.

4. Bake for 10 minutes, turning once. Allow to cool for 5 minutes before enjoying.

GLUTEN FREE ▪ DAIRY FREE ▪ LOW CALORIE

Nutrition Facts	
(amount per serving)	
Calories	244
Fat	22 g
Protein	6 g
Carbohydrate	8 g
Fiber	6 g

FIERY CHICKEN WINGS

These spicy and smoky chicken wings are sure to become a party favorite. They're especially good with cool and creamy Ranch Dip (page 208).

YIELD: 6 servings   PREP TIME: 5 minutes   COOK TIME: 30 minutes

⅓ cup coconut oil

¼ cup red wine vinegar

1 tablespoon ancho chile powder

¼ teaspoon ground cayenne pepper

1 teaspoon smoked paprika

2 cloves garlic

20 bone-in, skin-on chicken wings

sea salt

4 to 6 stalks celery

1. Preheat the oven to 375°F. Line a sheet pan with parchment paper.

2. To make the sauce, combine the oil, vinegar, spices, and garlic in a blender and puree until smooth. Season to taste with salt.

3. Place the sauce and chicken wings in a large bowl and toss to coat. Spread out on the sheet pan and roast for 30 minutes or until cooked through.

4. Allow to cool for at least 10 minutes, then serve with the celery stalks.

GLUTEN FREE · DAIRY FREE · LOW CALORIE

Nutrition Facts	
(amount per serving)	
Calories	437
Fat	31 g
Protein	36 g
Carbohydrate	3 g
Fiber	1.3 g

PARMESAN BAKED CHICKEN NUGGETS

These scrumptious nuggets are as tasty as the deep-fried version, but unlike the original, which contains 10 grams of carbs per serving, these have just 1 gram. Serve them with Ranch Dip (page 208) or Barbecue Sauce (page 212). I generally use freshly grated Parmesan, but go for the canned variety here, which has a texture more akin to breadcrumbs.

YIELD: 6 servings   PREP TIME: 10 minutes   COOK TIME: 16 to 18 minutes

4 boneless, skinless chicken thighs

¼ cup buttermilk

1 egg

1 cup grated Parmesan cheese

sea salt

freshly ground pepper

1. Preheat the oven to 400°F. Line a sheet pan with parchment paper.

2. Cut each of the chicken thighs into 3 pieces. Soak the chicken in the buttermilk for 10 minutes. Remove the chicken from the buttermilk and shake off any excess. Pat the chicken dry with paper towels.

3. In a medium bowl, whisk the egg and season with salt and pepper. Dip a piece of chicken into the egg, shaking off any excess, then dip into the Parmesan. Place the coated chicken onto the sheet pan and repeat with the remaining pieces of meat.

4. Bake for 16 to 18 minutes until the chicken is cooked through and the coating is beginning to brown.

GLUTEN FREE · LOW CALORIE

Nutrition Facts	
(amount per serving)	
Calories	217
Fat	12 g
Protein	25 g
Carbohydrate	1 g
Fiber	0 g

CRISPY BRUSSELS SPROUTS AND BACON

This recipe combines two polarizing ingredients—Brussels sprouts and bacon. One you may hate and the other you may love. I think after tasting these caramelized sprouts and chewy smoked bacon, even the most ardently opposed will fall in love with the cruciferous vegetable.

YIELD: 6 servings   PREP TIME: 10 minutes   COOK TIME: 30 to 35 minutes

1 pound Brussels sprouts, halved

2 tablespoons canola oil

4 slices thick-cut bacon, chopped into ½-inch pieces

sea salt

freshly ground pepper

1. Preheat the oven to 350°F.

2. Spread the Brussels sprouts over the sheet pan. Toss with the oil. Season with salt and pepper.

3. Sprinkle the bacon pieces over the Brussels sprouts.

4. Roast for 30 to 35 minutes or until the bacon has rendered its fat and the Brussels sprouts are browned on the bottoms.

GLUTEN FREE ▪ DAIRY FREE ▪ LOW CALORIE

Nutrition Facts	
(amount per serving)	
Calories	122
Fat	9 g
Protein	5 g
Carbohydrate	8 g
Fiber	3.2 g

MESQUITE STEAK AND VEGETABLE ROLLS

If you're tired of steak and vegetables on your ketogenic diet, here's a fun way to dress them up.

YIELD: 8 servings   PREP TIME: 10 minutes   COOK TIME: 25 minutes

2 teaspoons mesquite seasoning

2 tablespoons Worcestershire sauce

2 tablespoons canola oil

2 pounds skirt steak, sliced in 8 rectangular slices

1 small zucchini, cut into matchsticks, about 1 cup

1 medium red bell pepper, cut into thin slices

4 scallions, sliced lengthwise

sea salt

freshly ground pepper

1. Preheat the oven to 350°F.

2. Whisk the mesquite seasoning, Worcestershire sauce, and canola oil in a small bowl. Pour this over the skirt steak and season generously with salt and pepper.

3. Set a piece of steak on a cutting board with the short side facing you. Place a small handful of the zucchini, bell pepper, and scallions on the center of the steak and roll the steak away from you so that the vegetables stick out at each end. Secure with a toothpick.

4. Place the steak rolls on the sheet pan and bake for 25 minutes or until the steak is cooked through and the vegetables are crisp-tender.

GLUTEN FREE · DAIRY FREE · LOW CALORIE

Nutrition Facts	
(amount per serving)	
Calories	244
Fat	15 g
Protein	23 g
Carbohydrate	3 g
Fiber	0.8 g

COCONUT SHRIMP

Ubiquitous on appetizer menus, coconut shrimp is usually loaded with carbs thanks to breadcrumbs, sweetened coconut, and a sticky-sweet dipping sauce. This version uses a scant amount of coconut flour and shredded unsweetened coconut, along with a stevia-sweetened Thai Chili Sauce (page 215) for a much healthier option.

YIELD: 6 servings   PREP TIME: 5 minutes   COOK TIME: 7 to 10 minutes

1 pound jumbo shrimp, about 12

2 tablespoons coconut flour

1 teaspoon garlic powder

½ teaspoon sea salt

1 egg, whisked

½ cup shredded unsweetened coconut

1. Preheat the oven to 350°F. Line a sheet pan with parchment paper.

2. Peel and devein the shrimp, leaving the tails on. Slice the shrimp down the back, leaving it connected near the tail end. Fold each shrimp open, as if opening a book.

3. Combine the coconut flour, garlic powder, and salt in a shallow dish. Dip each shrimp into the coconut flour mixture to coat in a light dusting.

4. Dip the shrimp into the egg, shake off any excess, and then dip into the shredded coconut. Set the shrimp flat on the sheet pan.

5. Bake for 7 to 10 minutes until the shrimp are cooked through and the coconut begins to brown.

GLUTEN FREE · **DAIRY FREE** · **LOW CALORIE**

Nutrition Facts	
(amount per serving)	
Calories	148
Fat	7 g
Protein	18 g
Carbohydrate	4 g
Fiber	2.3 g

BACON-WRAPPED SCALLOPS

These decadent little flavor-bombs will be a hit at your next party. Or, transform them into a meal by serving them over steamed spinach with a splash of lemon juice and a drizzle of olive oil.

YIELD: 8 servings   PREP TIME: 10 minutes   COOK TIME: 10 minutes

16 slices bacon

1½ pounds large sea scallops, about 16

1 tablespoon olive oil

sea salt

freshly ground pepper

1. Preheat the oven to 400°F. Line a sheet pan with parchment paper.

2. Wrap each of the scallops with one slice of bacon. The bacon is longer than the circumference of the scallop and will overlap.

3. Brush the tops and bottoms of the scallops with oil. Place them on the sheet pan. Season with salt and pepper.

4. Bake for 10 minutes or until the scallops are cooked through and the bacon has rendered most of its fat.

GLUTEN FREE • DAIRY FREE • LOW CALORIE

Nutrition Facts	
(amount per serving)	
Calories	230
Fat	14 g
Protein	20 g
Carbohydrate	2 g
Fiber	0 g

CHAPTER FOUR

Vegetarian

Whether you're entertaining vegetarian guests or you simply want to take a break from meat for a meal or two, this chapter is filled with vegetarian and vegan ketogenic recipes. That might sound like an oxymoron, but it turns out there are plenty of low-carb, high-fat vegetarian foods, such as cheese, eggs, avocado, coconut, and nuts, to name a few.

SPINACH AND CHEESE-STUFFED PORTOBELLO MUSHROOMS

Portobello mushrooms are the perfect low-carb vessel for whatever you'd like to fill them with. This riff on spinach and cheese dip makes a delicious vegetarian dinner, or use smaller cremini mushrooms (also called "baby bella") and serve it as an appetizer.

YIELD: 4 servings   PREP TIME: 10 minutes   COOK TIME: 20 minutes

½ cup frozen spinach, defrosted

8 ounces cream cheese

8 ounces grated Parmesan cheese

1 teaspoon minced fresh rosemary

1 clove garlic, minced

4 portobello mushrooms, stems removed

sea salt

freshly ground pepper

1. Preheat the oven to 400°F.

2. Wring as much moisture as you can from the spinach.

3. Combine the spinach, cream cheese, Parmesan cheese, rosemary, and garlic in a small bowl. Season to taste with salt and pepper.

4. Place the mushrooms on the sheet pan and fill with the cheese mixture.

5. Bake for 20 minutes. Allow to cool for 5 minutes before serving.

GLUTEN FREE · VEGETARIAN · LOW CALORIE

Nutrition Facts	
(amount per serving)	
Calories	352
Fat	29 g
Protein	20 g
Carbohydrate	8 g
Fiber	1.9 g

CHEESY SPAGHETTI SQUASH BAKE

I was skeptical of spaghetti squash initially. I mean, how could a vege-table even come close to resembling real pasta? Then I tried it. While it's not exactly the same as wheat noodles, it comes close enough, especially when it's drowning in a sea of marinara sauce, melty cheese, and fresh basil.

YIELD: 4 servings   PREP TIME: 10 minutes   COOK TIME: 40 minutes

1 whole spaghetti squash, sliced into 1-inch-thick rounds and seeded

4 tablespoons olive oil, divided

1 cup Marinara Sauce (page 210) or store-bought, no-sugar-added marinara

8 ounces cream cheese, cut into 1-inch pieces

4 cups shredded Italian cheese blend

¼ cup thinly sliced fresh basil

1. Preheat the oven to 350°F. Line a sheet pan with parchment paper.

2. Spread the spaghetti squash rings out on the sheet pan and brush with 1 tablespoon of the oil, turning to coat on both sides.

3. Bake for 25 minutes. Remove the pan from the oven and allow to rest until cool enough to handle. Using a fork, shred the spaghetti squash strands into a large bowl.

4. Add the remaining 3 tablespoons of olive oil and the Marinara Sauce to the bowl. Toss gently to mix.

5. Fold the cream cheese into the spaghetti squash mixture.

6. Spread the spaghetti squash out onto the sheet pan and top with the Italian cheese blend. Return the pan to the oven and bake for 15 minutes or until the cheese is browned and bubbling.

7. Garnish with the fresh basil.

GLUTEN FREE ▪ VEGETARIAN

Nutrition Facts	
(amount per serving)	
Calories	601
Fat	52 g
Protein	26 g
Carbohydrate	14 g
Fiber	2 g

ROASTED RED PEPPER AND FONTINA PIZZA

I love the amazing flavor and convenience of jarred, roasted piquillo peppers. They are sweeter and more flavorful than bell peppers. But use whatever you have on hand. To make this recipe vegan, use an egg replacer and a nut- or soy-based vegan cheese in place of the Parmesan and fontina.

YIELD: 4 servings   PREP TIME: 20 minutes   COOK TIME: 20 to 22 minutes

1 medium head cauliflower, broken into florets

½ teaspoon sea salt

1 egg

½ cup grated Parmesan cheese

½ teaspoon garlic powder

¼ cup almond flour

¼ cup olive oil

1 cup roasted red peppers, thinly sliced

8 ounces fontina cheese, sliced

½ cup roughly chopped fresh basil

1. Preheat the oven to 425°F. Line a sheet pan with parchment paper.

2. Using the grater attachment on your food processor, grate the cauliflower. If you do not have a food processor, you can use a box grater, but it will take a while.

3. To prepare the cauliflower, spread it in a microwave-safe baking dish and microwave on high for 3 minutes. Stir and microwave again for 2 minutes. Set aside to cool for 10 minutes.

4. When the cauliflower is cool enough to handle, use your hands to squeeze as much of the moisture out of it as you can.

5. Thoroughly mix the cauliflower with the sea salt, egg, Parmesan cheese, garlic powder, and almond flour.

6. Press the mixture into the sheet pan in a circle, or spread it all the way to the edges for a thinner crust.

7. Bake for 12 minutes until the crust is beginning to brown.

8. Brush the top of the crust with olive oil and top with the red peppers and fontina. Bake for another 8 to 10 minutes or until the fontina is melted and beginning to brown. Shower the pizza with fresh basil.

GLUTEN FREE ▪ VEGETARIAN ▪ LOW CALORIE

Nutrition Facts	
(amount per serving)	
Calories	486
Fat	39 g
Protein	25 g
Carbohydrate	13 g
Fiber	4.8 g

FETA, OLIVE, AND SUN-DRIED TOMATO PIZZA

Feta cheese, olives, and spinach are delicious low-carb toppings for this vegetarian pie. The sun-dried tomatoes are optional. If you have carbs to spare, they add a sweet element that balances the briny olives and zesty cheese.

YIELD: 4 servings   PREP TIME: 15 minutes   COOK TIME: 17 minutes

1 medium head cauliflower, broken into florets

½ teaspoon sea salt

1 egg

½ cup grated Parmesan cheese

½ teaspoon garlic powder

1 teaspoon dried Italian herb blend (optional)

¼ cup almond flour

½ cup Marinara Sauce (page 210) or store-bought, no-sugar-added marinara

¼ cup pitted, halved Kalamata olives

¼ cup thinly sliced sun-dried tomatoes (optional)

8 ounces feta cheese, crumbled

2 cups roughly chopped baby spinach

1. Preheat the oven to 425°F. Line a sheet pan with parchment paper.

2. Using the grater attachment on your food processor, grate the cauliflower. If you do not have a food processor, you can use a box grater, but it will take a while.

3. To prepare the cauliflower, spread it in a microwave-safe baking dish and microwave on high for 3 minutes. Stir and microwave again for 2 minutes. Set aside to cool for 10 minutes.

4. When the cauliflower is cool enough to handle, use your hands to squeeze as much of the moisture out of it as you can.

5. Thoroughly mix the cauliflower with the sea salt, egg, Parmesan cheese, garlic powder, Italian herb blend (if using), and almond flour.

6. Press the mixture into the sheet pan in a circle, or spread it all the way to the edges for a thinner crust.

7. Bake for 12 minutes until the crust is lightly browned.

8. Brush the top of the crust with Marinara Sauce and top with the olives, sun-dried tomatoes (if using), and feta cheese. Bake for another 5 minutes or until the feta is beginning to brown. Shower the pizza with fresh spinach.

GLUTEN FREE ▪ VEGETARIAN ▪ LOW CALORIE

Nutrition Facts	
(amount per serving)	
Calories	365
Fat	25 g
Protein	20 g
Carbohydrate	18 g
Fiber	5.3 g

FOUR-CHEESE CALZONE

I developed the crust recipe for these mini calzones while working on another book devoted to gluten-free cooking and have adapted it to be lower carb for this book. You might be surprised to see sugar in the ingredient list, but don't worry, it feeds the yeast and doesn't contribute to the total carbs in the dish. If you prefer not to purchase the cheeses individually, opt for 16 ounces of an Italian cheese blend containing those listed.

YIELD: 6 servings   PREP TIME: 10 minutes   COOK TIME: 20 minutes

½ tablespoon sugar or honey

¼ cup hot water

1 package active-dry yeast, 2¼ teaspoons

1½ cups almond flour

½ cup tapioca starch

1 teaspoon sea salt

1 egg white

½ tablespoon apple cider vinegar

½ cup Marinara Sauce (page 210) or store-bought, no-sugar-added marinara

4 ounces shredded mozzarella cheese

4 ounces grated Parmesan cheese

4 ounces shredded fontina cheese

4 ounces grated Romano cheese

¼ cup minced fresh basil

1. Preheat the oven to 400°F. Line a sheet pan with parchment paper.

2. Dissolve the sugar into the hot water. When the water is about 110°F, sprinkle the yeast over the surface. Allow the mixture to rest for a few minutes until foamy.

3. Combine the almond meal, tapioca starch, and sea salt in a medium bowl. Make a well in the center and add the egg, vinegar, and yeast mixture. Stir to mix thoroughly.

4. Divide the dough into six pieces and place between two pieces of parchment paper. Use a rolling pin to roll each piece into a thin circle. Transfer the dough to the sheet pan.

5. Top each dough circle with a heaping tablespoon of Marinara Sauce and spread it out. Top each one with about 3 ounces of cheese and a little basil.

6. Fold the edges of each calzone together and crimp the edges.

7. Bake for 20 minutes until the crust is gently browned.

GLUTEN FREE · VEGETARIAN · LOW CALORIE

Nutrition Facts	
(amount per serving)	
Calories	454
Fat	32 g
Protein	27 g
Carbohydrate	18 g
Fiber	3.2 g

LASAGNA ZUCCHINI BOATS

Zucchini makes an excellent vehicle for, well, just about anything. Fill it with cheese, herbs, and marinara sauce for this riff on lasagna.

YIELD: 4 servings   PREP TIME: 10 minutes   COOK TIME: 20 to 25 minutes

4 medium zucchini, halved lengthwise

½ cup Marinara Sauce (page 210) or store-bought, no-sugar-added marinara

2 tablespoons minced shallots

4 cloves garlic, minced

2 cups ricotta cheese

1 egg, whisked

¼ cup minced fresh basil

½ cup grated Parmesan cheese

sea salt

freshly ground pepper

1. Preheat the oven to 400°F.

2. Scoop the flesh out of the zucchini using a small spoon. Leave about ¼ inch of flesh and skin so they hold up when baked. Spread about 1 tablespoon of the Marinara Sauce into each zucchini half.

3. In a small bowl, combine the shallots, garlic, ricotta, egg, and basil. Season with salt and pepper.

4. Divide the mixture between the zucchini and top each with 1 tablespoon of Parmesan.

5. Bake for 20 to 25 minutes or until the zucchini is soft and the cheese is browned and bubbling.

GLUTEN FREE • VEGETARIAN • LOW CALORIE

Nutrition Facts	
(amount per serving)	
Calories	332
Fat	21 g
Protein	22 g
Carbohydrate	14 g
Fiber	2.5 g

KUNG PAO CAULIFLOWER

The carbohydrate might seem high on this delicious vegan Chinese takeout recipe. But, with more than 6 grams of fiber, the net carbs drop dramatically. For more calories and protein, add marinated tofu, cut into 1-inch cubes.

YIELD: 4 servings   PREP TIME: 10 minutes   COOK TIME: 40 minutes

1 large head cauliflower, broken into florets

¼ cup coconut oil

2 teaspoons minced fresh ginger

2 teaspoons minced fresh garlic

¼ teaspoon red chile flakes

2 tablespoons low-sodium soy sauce

2 tablespoons balsamic vinegar

½ cup toasted cashews

2 scallions, sliced

sea salt

1. Preheat the oven to 375°F.

2. Toss the cauliflower with the coconut oil, ginger, garlic, and red chile flakes on the sheet pan. Season with salt.

3. Roast uncovered for 35 minutes or until the cauliflower is browned and slightly wilted.

4. Whisk together the soy sauce and vinegar. Pour the mixture over the roasted cauliflower and toss with the cashews and scallions. Roast for another 5 minutes.

GLUTEN FREE • VEGAN • DAIRY FREE • LOW CALORIE

Nutrition Facts	
(amount per serving)	
Calories	282
Fat	22 g
Protein	7 g
Carbohydrate	19 g
Fiber	6.1 g

ROASTED VEGETABLE FRITTATA

This easy frittata makes the perfect hands-off brunch dish or egg-based supper. It is also great for meal prep; leftovers can be covered and stored in the refrigerator for 2 to 3 days and reheated. Serve with Hollandaise Sauce (page 203) for an especially decadent meal.

YIELD: 4 servings   PREP TIME: 10 minutes   COOK TIME: 30 to 40 minutes

3 cups diced zucchini

2 cups diced onions

1 cup diced carrots

1 teaspoon minced fresh thyme

2 teaspoons minced fresh rosemary

¼ cup olive oil

1 dozen eggs

sea salt

freshly ground black pepper

1. Preheat the oven to 375°F.

2. Cut the vegetables into 1- to 2-inch pieces. Toss them with the herbs and olive oil on the sheet pan. Season with salt and pepper. Roast for 20 to 30 minutes or until soft and caramelized around the edges.

3. Combine the eggs in a large pitcher and whisk until nearly combined. Season with salt.

4. Pour the eggs into the sheet pan and return to the oven for 10 minutes or until the eggs are nearly set. Allow to rest for 5 minutes before cutting and serving.

GLUTEN FREE ▪ VEGETARIAN ▪ DAIRY FREE ▪ LOW CALORIE

Nutrition Facts	
(amount per serving)	
Calories	392
Fat	28 g
Protein	21 g
Carbohydrate	15 g
Fiber	4.3 g

ROASTED FENNEL AND ONION FRITTATA

Prepare the recipe for Roasted Vegetable Frittata but use 3 cups thinly sliced fennel bulb and 3 cups thinly sliced red onion in places of the other vegetables. Replace the herbs and olive oil with ¼ cup of softened Rosemary Orange Compound Butter (page 201).

GLUTEN FREE ▪ VEGETARIAN ▪ LOW CALORIE

Nutrition Facts	
(amount per serving)	
Calories	384
Fat	26 g
Protein	21 g
Carbohydrate	16 g
Fiber	4.2 g

BAKED EGGPLANT STACKS

Roasting eggplant makes it sweet, soft, and caramelized—far more flavorful than the traditional pasta dough used in making lasagna and other layered pasta dishes. To make this vegan, use a homemade ricotta nut-cheese; see variation.

YIELD: 4 servings   PREP TIME: 10 minutes   COOK TIME: 30 to 35 minutes

1 medium eggplant, sliced in 12 slices

¼ cup olive oil

4 cloves garlic, minced

1 cup Marinara Sauce (page 210) or store-bought, no-sugar-added marinara

2 cups ricotta cheese

sea salt

freshly ground pepper

1. Preheat the oven to 375°F.

2. Spread the eggplant out on a sheet pan. Pour the olive oil over the eggplant and turn to coat. Sprinkle the garlic over the slices and season with salt and pepper.

3. Bake for 20 minutes until the eggplant is soft and beginning to brown.

4. Remove the sheet pan from the oven. Turn the eggplant slices over, then top four of them with 2 tablespoons Marinara Sauce and ¼ cup of ricotta cheese. Top with another eggplant slice, followed by more marinara and ricotta. Finish with a final slice of eggplant.

5. Bake the eggplant stacks for 10 to 15 minutes or until the ricotta is warmed.

GLUTEN FREE • VEGETARIAN • LOW CALORIE

Nutrition Facts	
(amount per serving)	
Calories	390
Fat	30 g
Protein	16 g
Carbohydrate	16 g
Fiber	3.9 g

VEGAN EGGPLANT STACKS WITH MACADAMIA CHEESE

Prepare the Baked Eggplant Stacks but instead of the ricotta cheese, make a macadamia cheese. Blend 1 cup macadamia nuts, soaked overnight, with 1 garlic clove, 1 tablespoon nutritional yeast, 2 tablespoons extra-virgin olive oil, 1 tablespoon lemon juice, and ⅓ to ½ cup water, as needed to blend.

GLUTEN FREE ▪ VEGETARIAN ▪ DAIRY FREE ▪ LOW CALORIE

Nutrition Facts	
(amount per serving)	
Calories	476
Fat	46 g
Protein	5 g
Carbohydrate	17 g
Fiber	6.8 g

BROCCOLI AND TOFU SPAGHETTI SQUASH NOODLE BOWL

A similar recipe also appears in the poultry chapter, but it is just as flavorful using marinated tofu for a vegan entrée. Use gluten-free soy sauce for a gluten-free version.

YIELD: 4 servings   PREP TIME: 10 minutes   COOK TIME: 30 minutes

16 ounces extra-firm tofu

1 tablespoon sesame oil

⅓ cup soy sauce

2 tablespoons lime juice

1 teaspoon minced fresh garlic

1 teaspoon minced fresh ginger

1 small spaghetti squash, about 1½ pounds

2 cups broccoli florets

2 cups halved button mushrooms

1 tablespoon olive oil

1. Preheat the oven to 375°F. Line a sheet pan with parchment paper.

2. Slice the tofu in half horizontally and press it between two cutting boards or plates to remove some of the liquid.

3. Whisk the sesame oil, soy sauce, lime juice, garlic, and ginger in a shallow dish. Place the pressed tofu into the dish and turn to coat. Allow it to marinate for 5 minutes.

4. Slice the spaghetti squash into 1-inch-thick rings and use a paring knife to remove the seeds and strings. Spread the rings on the sheet pan.

5. Spread the broccoli and mushrooms onto the pan around the spaghetti squash and drizzle with the olive oil. Season with salt and pepper.

6. Slice the tofu into 1-inch cubes and add them to the pan on top of and around the broccoli, reserving the remaining marinade. Bake for 30 minutes.

7. Remove the pan from the oven and transfer the spaghetti squash to a cutting board.

8. Pour the sesame dressing over the tofu and vegetables, tossing gently to coat.

9. Use a fork to shred the spaghetti squash into long, thin strands. Oven mitts are helpful because the squash will still be hot.

10. Divide the spaghetti squash between four serving bowls. Top with the tofu and vegetables, making sure to get some of the sauce.

GLUTEN FREE · VEGETARIAN · DAIRY FREE · LOW CALORIE

Nutrition Facts	
(amount per serving)	
Calories	213
Fat	13 g
Protein	15 g
Carbohydrate	15 g
Fiber	4.6 g

ROASTED PEPPERCORN TOFU AND BROCCOLINI

My husband Rich is a vegetarian, so I'm always eager to find yummy meatless recipes he can enjoy. This oven-roasted tofu and broccoli is loaded with flavor from complex black peppercorns, savory minced ginger, and spicy chili paste. The recipe serves a small portion for four or a generous serving for two. Even the larger portion yields just 13 grams of net carbs.

YIELD: 4 servings   PREP TIME: 10 minutes   COOK TIME: 25 minutes

1 teaspoon whole black peppercorns

1 tablespoon minced garlic

1 tablespoon minced ginger

1 tablespoon soy sauce

1 teaspoon chili paste, such as sambal oelek

3 tablespoons canola oil

16 ounces extra-firm tofu, drained and cut into 1-inch cubes

2 bunches broccolini

1 tablespoon toasted sesame oil

1 tablespoon sesame seeds

2 scallions, thinly sliced

1. Preheat the oven to 400°F.

2. Toast the black peppercorns in a dry skillet over medium heat until fragrant, about 2 minutes. Grind in a pepper grinder or mortar and pestle.

3. In a medium bowl, combine the ground peppercorns with the garlic, ginger, soy sauce, chili paste, and canola oil. Add the tofu and stir gently to coat it in the marinade.

4. Spread the broccolini onto a sheet pan and toss with the sesame oil. Season with salt and pepper.

5. Add the marinated tofu to the pan.

6. Bake for 25 minutes or until the broccolini is tender and beginning to brown around the edges.

7. Sprinkle with sesame seeds and scallions before serving.

VEGETARIAN ▪ DAIRY FREE ▪ LOW CALORIE

Nutrition Facts	
(amount per serving)	
Calories	250
Fat	19 g
Protein	13 g
Carbohydrate	13 g
Fiber	6.1 g

COCONUT-CRUSTED TOFU WITH HONEY MUSTARD SAUCE

After years of pan-frying tofu, I found this method for oven baking. It is easy and yields a deliciously crispy exterior. You can take the tofu in myriad directions—tacos, dipped in Thai Chili Sauce (page 215), or with this easy take on honey mustard sauce.

YIELD: 4 servings PREP TIME: 5 minutes COOK TIME: 15 minutes

1 block extra-firm tofu, 14 to 16 ounces

6 tablespoons canola oil, divided

½ cup shredded unsweetened coconut

2 tablespoons apple cider vinegar

1 teaspoon Dijon mustard

4 to 6 drops liquid stevia

1. Preheat the oven to 400°F.

2. Slice the tofu in half horizontally so that you have two flat rectangles. Place them between two cutting boards and place a heavy object, such as a cast-iron skillet, on top of the top board. You may wish to line the cutting boards with paper towels to soak up some of the moisture. Press for at least 5 minutes.

3. Slice each of the pressed tofu pieces into 4 strips.

4. Coat the tofu in 2 tablespoons of the canola oil. Sprinkle with the coconut and toss gently to coat.

5. Spread the tofu on the sheet pan and bake for 15 minutes.

6. Meanwhile, whisk the remaining 4 tablespoons of canola oil with the apple cider vinegar, Dijon mustard, and liquid stevia, to taste. Whisk until emulsified.

7. Allow the tofu to cool for 5 minutes or until you can pick it up without burning your fingers. Serve it with the honey mustard sauce.

GLUTEN FREE ▪ VEGETARIAN ▪ DAIRY FREE ▪ LOW CALORIE

Nutrition Facts	
(amount per serving)	
Calories	308
Fat	30 g
Protein	11 g
Carbohydrate	3 g
Fiber	1.8 g

ROSEMARY PECAN TOFU CUTLETS

Rosemary, toasted pecans, and sea salt form a tasty crust for these cutlets, which are delicious served with Mashed Cauliflower (page 221).

YIELD: 4 servings   PREP TIME: 5 minutes   COOK TIME: 15 minutes

1 block extra-firm tofu, 14 to 16 ounces

2 tablespoons canola oil, divided

½ cup ground toasted pecans

1 teaspoon minced rosemary

½ teaspoon sea salt

¼ teaspoon freshly ground pepper

1. Preheat the oven to 400°F.

2. Slice the tofu in half horizontally so that you have two flat rectangles. Place them between two cutting boards and place a heavy object, such as a cast-iron skillet, on top of the top board. You may wish to line the cutting boards with paper towels to soak up some of the moisture. Press for at least 5 minutes.

3. Slice each of the pressed tofu pieces into 4 strips.

4. Coat the tofu in 2 tablespoons of the canola oil.

5. Combine the pecans, rosemary, sea salt, and pepper in a small bowl. Sprinkle this mixture over the tofu and toss gently to coat.

6. Spread the tofu on the sheet pan and bake for 15 minutes.

GLUTEN FREE ▪ VEGETARIAN ▪ DAIRY FREE ▪ LOW CALORIE

Nutrition Facts	
(amount per serving)	
Calories	253
Fat	23 g
Protein	12 g
Carbohydrate	4 g
Fiber	2.6 g

STUFFED EGGPLANT WITH FETA AND PINE NUTS

Eggplant is one of my favorite vegetables. It is especially good when it is roasted in the oven until meltingly tender. In this recipe, it's first roasted and then stuffed with feta, minced shallots, garlic, and parsley before another stint in the oven.

YIELD: 4 servings   PREP TIME: 5 minutes   COOK TIME: 50 minutes

1 eggplant, sliced in half lengthwise

¼ cup olive oil

12 ounces feta cheese, crumbled

2 tablespoons minced shallots

2 teaspoons minced garlic

½ cup fresh parsley

sea salt

freshly ground pepper

1. Preheat the oven to 425°F.

2. Place the eggplant skin-side down on a sheet pan. Brush with olive oil and season generously with salt. Bake for 30 minutes.

3. In a medium bowl, combine feta, shallots, garlic, and parsley. Season with salt and pepper.

4. Spoon the feta mixture over the eggplants. Bake for 20 minutes until the eggplants are tender and the feta is beginning to brown. Allow to rest for 5 minutes before serving. Slice each eggplant half in half again to serve.

GLUTEN FREE · VEGETARIAN · LOW CALORIE

Nutrition Facts	
(amount per serving)	
Calories	434
Fat	36 g
Protein	15 g
Carbohydrate	15 g
Fiber	4.3 g

TERIYAKI TEMPEH SKEWERS

Sweet and spicy teriyaki sauce cuts through some of the bitterness of tempeh. Serve this with Savoy Cabbage and Almond Slaw (page 217).

YIELD: 4 servings   PREP TIME: 5 minutes   COOK TIME: 25 minutes

16 ounces tempeh, cut into 2-inch pieces

2 tablespoons canola oil

½ cup Teriyaki Sauce (page 214)

sea salt

freshly ground black pepper

1. Preheat the oven to 400°F. Line a sheet pan with parchment paper.

2. Thread the tempeh onto skewers and brush with the oil. Season with salt and pepper. Bake for 15 minutes.

3. Brush the Teriyaki Sauce onto the tempeh and return to the oven for another 10 minutes until the sauce is bubbling and sticky.

GLUTEN FREE ▪ **VEGETARIAN** ▪ **DAIRY FREE** ▪ **LOW CALORIE**

Nutrition Facts	
(amount per serving)	
Calories	278
Fat	17 g
Protein	24 g
Carbohydrate	12 g
Fiber	6 g

BARBECUE TEMPEH WITH WILTED SPINACH

Prepare the Teriyaki Tempeh Skewers but use Barbecue Sauce (page 212) in place of the Teriyaki Sauce. Mix 4 cups spinach with 2 tablespoons olive oil and 1 clove minced garlic, and add to the sheet pan during the last 5 minutes of cooking. Serve with Mashed Cauliflower (page 221).

GLUTEN FREE ▪ VEGETARIAN ▪ DAIRY FREE ▪ LOW CALORIE

Nutrition Facts	
(amount per serving)	
Calories	335
Fat	24 g
Protein	21 g
Carbohydrate	11 g
Fiber	6.8 g

CHAPTER FIVE

Seafood

I live in sunny Southern California where fresh seafood abounds, but if you're landlocked, look no further than the frozen case. The fish is fresher this way because it is flash-frozen on the boat and isn't defrosted until it reaches your kitchen. In this chapter, I share some of my favorite recipes for fish and seafood. I'm a particular fan of salmon, which is rich in fat and a favorite in the Northwest, where I grew up.

SALSA VERDE SHRIMP

Enjoy these shrimp as a filling for low-carb wraps or served over Cauliflower Rice (page 220).

YIELD: 2 servings   PREP TIME: 10 minutes   COOK TIME: 5 to 7 minutes

1 pound large shrimp, peeled and deveined

1 cup Salsa Verde (page 207)

½ small red onion, thinly sliced

1 tablespoon red wine vinegar

handful fresh cilantro

1. Preheat the oven to 400°F. Line a sheet pan with parchment paper.

2. Toss the shrimp with the Salsa Verde and spread out on the sheet pan.

3. Bake for 5 to 7 minutes or until the shrimp are cooked through.

4. Meanwhile, combine the red onion and red wine vinegar in a small bowl. Set aside.

5. Toss the cooked shrimp with the marinated onion and fresh cilantro.

GLUTEN FREE · DAIRY FREE · LOW CALORIE

Nutrition Facts	
(amount per serving)	
Calories	498
Fat	32 g
Protein	46 g
Carbohydrate	8 g
Fiber	0.6 g

SHRIMP FAJITA BOWLS

Enjoy these roasted vegetables and spicy shrimp over shredded cabbage and topped with fresh cilantro, homemade guacamole, and sour cream. It's a delicious low-carb meal with the perfect balance of flavors and textures.

YIELD: 4 servings   PREP TIME: 10 minutes   COOK TIME: 30 minutes

1 medium green bell pepper, cored and thinly sliced

1 medium red bell pepper, cored and thinly sliced

1 medium yellow onion, halved and sliced

2 tablespoons canola oil, divided

3 teaspoons chili powder, divided

1 pound large shrimp, peeled and deveined

1 tablespoon lime juice

sea salt

freshly ground pepper

1 large clove garlic, minced

1 cup shredded green cabbage

½ cup roughly chopped fresh cilantro

½ cup Guacamole (page 206)

½ cup sour cream

1. Preheat the oven to 400°F.

2. Spread the bell peppers and onion on a sheet pan and toss with 1 tablespoon of the oil. Sprinkle the vegetables with 1 teaspoon of the chili powder and season with salt and pepper. Toss to mix. Roast for 20 minutes.

3. While the vegetables cook, toss the shrimp in the remaining table-spoon of oil, 2 teaspoons of chili powder, and lime juice. Add the garlic. Allow to marinate.

4. Remove the pan from the oven and spread the shrimp and mar-inade onto the sheet pan. Bake for 10 minutes or until the shrimp is cooked through.

5. To serve, combine the cabbage and cilantro in a small bowl and top with the roasted peppers and shrimp. Top with Guacamole and sour cream.

GLUTEN FREE ▪ LOW CALORIE

Nutrition Facts	
(amount per serving)	
Calories	324
Fat	19 g
Protein	25 g
Carbohydrate	13 g
Fiber	4.3 g

PRAWNS PROVENÇAL

The roasted vegetables and herbs in this recipe remind me of rata-touille. Choose large prawns for this recipe, about 8 or 10 per pound if possible.

YIELD: 4 servings   PREP TIME: 10 minutes   COOK TIME: 37 to 39 minutes

1 large zucchini, cut into 1-inch pieces

1 medium yellow onion, diced

2 cloves garlic, roughly chopped

8 ounces grape tomatoes

1 small to medium eggplant, cut into ½-inch pieces

1 teaspoon minced fresh thyme

1 teaspoon anchovy paste

¼ cup olive oil

1 pound jumbo prawns, peeled and deveined

2 sprigs fresh basil, minced

sea salt

freshly ground pepper

1. Preheat the oven to 375°F. Line a sheet pan with parchment paper.

2. Spread the zucchini, onion, garlic, grape tomatoes, eggplant, and thyme on the sheet pan.

3. Whisk the anchovy paste into the olive oil and pour it over the vegetables. Toss gently to coat. Season with salt and pepper.

4. Roast for 30 minutes until the vegetables are very soft and beginning to brown.

5. Add the prawns to the vegetables and return the pan to the oven just until the prawns are cooked through, about 7 to 9 minutes. Sprinkle with the fresh basil before serving.

GLUTEN FREE · DAIRY FREE · LOW CALORIE

Nutrition Facts	
(amount per serving)	
Calories	352
Fat	20 g
Protein	25 g
Carbohydrate	18 g
Fiber	4.4 g

BUTTERY LIME-BAKED HALIBUT AND SCALLIONS

This simple, low-carb baked fish is rich and buttery with a balanced tang from the limes and a mellow bite from the roasted scallions, also called green onions. Here I serve it over a bed of arugula, but use another delicate leafy green if you prefer.

YIELD: 4 servings   PREP TIME: 10 minutes   COOK TIME: 15 to 18 minutes

1 lime

3 scallions, divided

1 stick (½ cup) butter, softened

4 halibut filets, about 5 ounces each

sea salt

freshly ground pepper

4 cups loosely packed arugula

1. Preheat the oven to 400°F. Line a sheet pan with parchment paper.

2. Zest the lime using a Microplane grater. Mince one of the scallions. Combine the lime zest, scallions, and butter in a small bowl.

3. Coat the fish in the butter mixture and set on the sheet pan. Season with salt and pepper.

4. Thinly slice the lime and spread it over the fish filets.

5. Slice the remaining 2 scallions in half lengthwise and lay them on the sheet pan.

6. Bake for 15 to 18 minutes until the halibut is cooked through and flakes easily with a fork.

7. To serve, divide the arugula among serving plates and spoon some of the pan juices over them. Top with a halibut filet and garnish with 1 piece of scallion.

GLUTEN FREE · DAIRY FREE · LOW CALORIE

Nutrition Facts	
(amount per serving)	
Calories	429
Fat	28 g
Protein	38 g
Carbohydrate	4 g
Fiber	1 g

SOY GINGER SALMON WITH ROASTED MUSHROOMS

Toasted sesame oil and spicy ginger add complexity to this otherwise very simple dish.

YIELD: 4 servings   PREP TIME: 10 minutes   COOK TIME: 17 to 20 minutes

2 cups halved mushrooms	1 tablespoon minced fresh ginger
1 green bell pepper, cored and cut into 1-inch pieces	1 pound salmon, cut into four 4-ounce filets
3 tablespoons toasted sesame oil, divided	sea salt
1 tablespoon soy sauce	freshly ground pepper
zest and juice of 1 lime	1 tablespoon sesame seeds

1. Preheat the oven to 400°F. Line a sheet pan with parchment paper.

2. Spread the mushrooms and bell pepper on the sheet pan. Drizzle with 1 tablespoon of the toasted sesame oil and season with salt and pepper. Roast for 10 minutes.

3. Meanwhile, whisk together the remaining 2 tablespoons of sesame oil, soy sauce, lime zest and juice, and ginger in a small bowl. Brush this mixture over the salmon filets, turning to coat.

4. Reduce the heat to 325°F. Make room on the pan for the salmon filets and add them to the pan.

5. Roast for 7 to 10 minutes until the salmon is opaque on the outside and flakes easily with a fork but is still deep pink on the inside.

6. To serve, sprinkle with the sesame seeds.

GLUTEN FREE · DAIRY FREE · LOW CALORIE

Nutrition Facts	
(amount per serving)	
Calories	294
Fat	17 g
Protein	31 g
Carbohydrate	5 g
Fiber	1.4 g

BAKED SALMON WITH HONEY MUSTARD CREAM SAUCE

This slow-roasted salmon is bathed in a luxurious honey mustard cream sauce. Swap the broccolini for broccoli or asparagus if you prefer. Serve with a simple side salad. If you purchase salmon with the skin on, you can remove the skin with ease after baking by sliding a metal spatula between the fish and the skin.

YIELD: 4 servings   PREP TIME: 5 minutes   COOK TIME: 23 to 24 minutes

1 pound broccolini	2 teaspoons Dijon mustard
2 tablespoons olive oil	⅓ cup heavy cream
1 pound salmon filet	sea salt
1 teaspoon honey	freshly ground pepper

1. Preheat the oven to 225°F. Line a sheet pan with parchment paper.

2. Toss the broccolini with the olive oil and spread it around the edges of the sheet pan, leaving space in the center. Season with salt and pepper.

3. Bake for 10 minutes. Remove the pan from the oven.

4. Place the salmon in the center of the sheet pan and season with salt and pepper.

5. Bake for 10 minutes until the salmon is just beginning to become opaque around the edges.

6. Whisk the honey, mustard, and heavy cream in a small measuring cup. Pour the mixture over the salmon and return the pan to the oven to cook for another 3 to 4 minutes or until the salmon flakes easily with a fork but is still a deeper color of pink in the center. It will continue to cook a bit in the seconds after coming out of the oven.

GLUTEN FREE • LOW CALORIE

Nutrition Facts
(amount per serving)

Calories	340
Fat	22 g
Protein	26 g
Carbohydrate	10 g
Fiber	3.1 g

SALMON AND FENNEL WITH ORANGE

The simplicity of this dish does not convey the depth of flavor. The long, slow cooking time caramelizes the fennel and renders the orange slices chewy and delectable. It is one of my favorite weeknight suppers.

YIELD: 4 servings   PREP TIME: 10 minutes   COOK TIME: 27 to 30 minutes

1 fennel bulb, thinly sliced in 12 to 16 wedges, fronds reserved

1 orange, unpeeled, thinly sliced

¼ cup olive oil

1½ to 2-pound salmon filet

sea salt

freshly ground pepper

1. Preheat the oven to 400°F.

2. Spread the fennel wedges and orange slices on the sheet pan. Drizzle with the olive oil and season with salt. Roast for 15 minutes.

3. Remove the pan from the oven and reduce the oven temperature to 225°F.

4. Turn the fennel and orange slices over. Make space for the salmon in the center of the pan.

5. Return the pan to the oven and roast for another 12 to 15 minutes or until the salmon is opaque and begins to render white along the edges. The center should flake with a fork and be a darker shade of pink on the inside.

6. The salmon will continue to cook in the time it takes to remove it from the pan and serve. Season the salmon with salt and pepper before serving.

GLUTEN FREE · DAIRY FREE · LOW CALORIE

Nutrition Facts	
(amount per serving)	
Calories	493
Fat	34 g
Protein	38 g
Carbohydrate	8 g
Fiber	2.6 g

HALIBUT WITH TARRAGON COMPOUND BUTTER AND GREEN BEANS

Cooking in parchment keeps the halibut nice and tender while it cooks and helps the green beans cook in a moist heat. Choose thin French green beans for a delicate texture and flavor. If you prefer to keep this super simple, replace the Tarragon Compound Butter with a store-bought compound butter.

YIELD: 4 servings   PREP TIME: 10 minutes   COOK TIME: 15 minutes

8 ounces green beans, trimmed

1 stick (½ cup) Tarragon Compound Butter (page 202)

4 halibut filets, about 4 ounces each

sea salt

freshly ground pepper

1. Preheat the oven to 400°F. Cut four large squares of parchment paper.

2. Divide the green beans between the parchment squares. Top each bundle with 1 tablespoon of the compound butter.

3. Set the halibut filets on top of the green beans, season with salt and pepper, and top with another tablespoon of the compound butter.

4. Seal the packages by bringing the sides of the parchment together and then folding them, as if folding a paper lunch sack. Fold the ends underneath.

5. Bake for 15 minutes, or until the halibut flakes easily with a fork and the green beans are crisp and tender.

GLUTEN FREE · DAIRY FREE · LOW CALORIE

Nutrition Facts	
(amount per serving)	
Calories	381
Fat	26 g
Protein	32 g
Carbohydrate	5 g
Fiber	2.1 g

BACON-WRAPPED SHRIMP

Avoid thick-cut bacon for this recipe. The thinner slices will cook at the same rate as the shrimp and be done at the same time. The meal is delicious on its own or paired with Mashed Cauliflower (page 221).

YIELD: 4 servings   PREP TIME: 10 minutes   COOK TIME: 10 to 12 minutes

2 pounds extra-jumbo shrimp, about 10 to 12 per pound, peeled and deveined

10 to 12 slices bacon, each cut into two shorter strips

1 teaspoon minced rosemary

freshly ground pepper

1. Preheat the oven to 450°F. Line a sheet pan with parchment paper.

2. Wrap each piece of shrimp in a half slice of bacon and place seam-side down on the sheet pan.

3. Season with rosemary and pepper.

4. Bake for 10 to 12 minutes or until the bacon is beginning to crisp and the shrimp are cooked through.

GLUTEN FREE ▪ DAIRY FREE ▪ LOW CALORIE

Nutrition Facts	
(amount per serving)	
Calories	416
Fat	19 g
Protein	54 g
Carbohydrate	2 g
Fiber	0 g

SAUSAGE, SHRIMP, AND BOK CHOY

This recipe draws from a couple global cuisines. With sausage and seafood, it gives a nod to paella. But add the bok choy, and it suddenly feels like a stir-fry. Whatever you call it, it's just delicious! The sausage infuses the bok choy and shrimp with flavor.

YIELD: 4 servings   PREP TIME: 10 minutes   COOK TIME: 15 to 20 minutes

4 pork sausage links, cut into 1-inch pieces

1 pound large shrimp, about 10 to 15 per pound, peeled and deveined

4 heads baby bok choy, halved lengthwise

¼ cup olive oil

sea salt

freshly ground pepper

1. Preheat the oven to 350°F. Line a sheet pan with parchment paper.

2. Spread the sausage, shrimp, and bok choy onto the sheet pan. Drizzle with the olive oil. Toss gently to coat, turning the bok choy so that it is cut-side down on the sheet pan. Season with salt and pepper.

3. Bake for 15 to 20 minutes or until the sausage is cooked through.

GLUTEN FREE · DAIRY FREE · LOW CALORIE

Nutrition Facts	
(amount per serving)	
Calories	536
Fat	39 g
Protein	41 g
Carbohydrate	4 g
Fiber	0.1 g

CLASSIC CRAB CAKES WITH LEMON SOUR CREAM

The trick to making low-carb crab cakes is baking them in the oven instead of pan-frying them. They hold together until the egg sets and binds all of the ingredients. The coconut flour helps absorb excess moisture as they bake.

YIELD: 4 servings   PREP TIME: 5 minutes   COOK TIME: 15 minutes

1 egg

1½ tablespoons coconut flour

1 tablespoon Old Bay seasoning

16 ounces lump crab meat, picked over for shells

1 scallion, white and green parts, thinly sliced

1 tablespoon canola oil

1 cup full-fat sour cream

½ cup mayonnaise

1 teaspoon minced fresh dill

zest and juice of 1 lemon

1. Preheat the oven to 400°F. Line a sheet pan with parchment paper.

2. In a medium bowl, whisk the egg, coconut flour, and Old Bay seasoning. Fold in the crabmeat and scallion.

3. Form the mixture into 8 small cakes and place them on the sheet pan. Brush gently with the canola oil.

4. Bake for 15 minutes or until the cakes are set and beginning to brown around the edges. Transfer to individual serving plates.

5. While the crab cakes bake, whisk the sour cream, mayonnaise, dill, lemon zest, and lemon juice in a small bowl.

6. To serve, plate the crab cakes and top them with the lemon sour cream.

GLUTEN FREE • LOW CALORIE

Nutrition Facts	
(amount per serving)	
Calories	489
Fat	38 g
Protein	30 g
Carbohydrate	6 g
Fiber	1.6 g

ASIAN CRAB CAKES WITH SRIRACHA MAYO

Spice up basic crab cakes with a little ginger, garlic, and sriracha.

YIELD: 4 servings   PREP TIME: 5 minutes   COOK TIME: 15 minutes

1 egg

1½ tablespoons coconut flour

2 teaspoons minced ginger

2 cloves garlic, minced

½ teaspoon sea salt

½ teaspoon freshly ground pepper

16 ounces lump crab meat, picked over for shells

2 tablespoons roughly chopped fresh cilantro

2 tablespoons canola oil

½ cup mayonnaise

zest and juice of 1 lime

2 teaspoons sriracha

1. Preheat the oven to 400°F. Line a sheet pan with parchment paper.

2. In a medium bowl, whisk the egg, coconut flour, ginger, garlic, salt, and pepper. Fold in the crabmeat and cilantro.

3. Form the mixture into 8 small cakes and place them on the sheet pan. Brush gently with the canola oil.

4. Bake for 15 minutes or until the cakes are set and beginning to brown around the edges. Transfer to individual serving plates.

5. While the crab cakes bake, whisk the mayonnaise, lime zest, lime juice, and sriracha in a small bowl. Drizzle the sriracha mayo over the crab cakes.

GLUTEN FREE · LOW CALORIE

Nutrition Facts	
(amount per serving)	
Calories	373
Fat	26 g
Protein	28 g
Carbohydrate	5 g
Fiber	1.8 g

CHAPTER SIX

Poultry

Poultry is a meal standby in my kitchen, as I imagine it is in yours. I often purchase whole birds to save money and enjoy richer cuts of meat, not to mention the bones, which make an excellent stock. It's also nice to keep a bag of frozen chicken breasts or thighs in the freezer to defrost at a moment's notice. To keep fat high and protein in moderation, use bone-in, skin-on chicken thighs and drumsticks. This chapter includes a mixture of breasts, thighs, drumsticks, and whole chicken.

CHICKEN CHILE RELLENO

This is an inside-out version of the battered, pan-fried Mexican cuisine classic. It has all the flavor of the original, with only 1 gram of net carbs! Serve with Salsa Verde (page 207) and Cauliflower Rice (page 220).

YIELD: 4 servings   PREP TIME: 5 minutes   COOK TIME: 25 minutes

4 boneless, skinless chicken breasts

2 whole green poblano chiles

4 ounces queso fresco

¼ cup almond meal

1 tablespoon ground cumin

1 tablespoon smoked paprika

½ teaspoon sea salt

¼ teaspoon freshly ground black pepper

1 egg, whisked

1. Preheat the oven to 400°F.

2. Pound the chicken breasts to about ¼-inch thickness between two sheets of parchment paper using the flat side of a meat cleaver.

3. Slice the green chiles in half and place one half on each of the chicken breasts. Top each with 1 ounce of queso fresco, about 2 tablespoons.

4. Roll each of the chicken breasts into a tight cylinder and secure with a toothpick.

5. On a plate, combine the almond meal, cumin, paprika, sea salt, and pepper.

6. Carefully dip each of the chicken rolls into the whisked egg and then dredge in the almond flour mixture. Place the chicken on the sheet pan, seam-side down.

7. Bake for 25 minutes or until the chicken is cooked through and beginning to brown.

GLUTEN FREE · LOW CALORIE

Nutrition Facts
(amount per serving)

Calories	347
Fat	15 g
Protein	48 g
Carbohydrate	2 g
Fiber	1 g

CHICKEN ENCHILADA ZUCCHINI BOATS

Transform leftovers into these flavorful low-carb enchiladas. Use store-bought rotisserie chicken or meat from a Basic Roasted Chicken (page 120).

YIELD: 4 servings   PREP TIME: 5 minutes   COOK TIME: 20 to 25 minutes

8 small zucchini, halved lengthwise

2 cups shredded cooked chicken (about 1 pound)

1 cup Enchilada Sauce (page 211), or 1 can store-bought

2 cups shredded Mexican-blend cheese, divided

½ cup full-fat sour cream

1. Preheat the oven to 400°F.

2. Scoop most of the flesh out of the zucchini and reserve for another use. Leave enough of the skin and flesh so that it doesn't collapse, about ⅛-inch thickness.

3. Combine the chicken, Enchilada Sauce, and 1 cup of the shredded cheese in a large bowl. Mix to combine.

4. Divide the mixture between the zucchini halves and place them on a sheet pan. Top each with the remaining shredded cheese, pressing it down to keep it from falling out.

5. Bake for 20 to 25 minutes until the zucchini are soft and the cheese is browned and bubbling.

6. Top with the sour cream to serve.

GLUTEN FREE · LOW CALORIE

Nutrition Facts	
(amount per serving)	
Calories	496
Fat	31 g
Protein	42 g
Carbohydrate	13 g
Fiber	3.1 g

CAPRESE CHICKEN

Caprese salad meets baked chicken in this easy one-pan dinner. Make sure to use a fresh, vine-ripened tomato and fresh basil for the best flavor. Bake with Prosciutto-Wrapped Asparagus (page 42) for a complete meal.

YIELD: 4 servings   PREP TIME: 15 minutes to 8 hours
COOK TIME: 25 minutes

4 boneless, skinless chicken breasts

¼ cup balsamic vinegar

2 tablespoons olive oil

½ teaspoon sea salt, plus more to taste

¼ teaspoon freshly ground black pepper, plus more to taste

1 vine-ripened tomato, sliced in 8 thin slices

4 ounces fresh mozzarella cheese, sliced in ⅛-inch-thick slices

¼ cup minced fresh basil

1. Preheat the oven to 400°F.

2. Pound the chicken breasts to about ¼-inch thickness between two sheets of parchment paper using a meat cleaver.

3. Whisk the balsamic vinegar, olive oil, sea salt, and pepper and coat the chicken breasts in this mixture. Marinate for at least 10 minutes while you prepare the other ingredients. If you have time, allow the chicken to marinate in the balsamic mixture in the refrigerator for up to 8 hours.

4. Remove the chicken from the marinade and shake off any excess liquid.

5. Place the chicken on the sheet pan. Place 2 slices of the tomato on top of each of the chicken breasts. Top each one with 2 slices of mozzarella and 1 tablespoon minced basil. Season with salt and pepper.

6. Bake for 25 minutes or until the chicken is cooked through and the cheese is browned and bubbling.

GLUTEN FREE ▪ LOW CALORIE

Nutrition Facts (amount per serving)	
Calories	365
Fat	18 g
Protein	45 g
Carbohydrate	4 g
Fiber	0.4 g

CHICKEN THIGHS WITH BACON MUSTARD CREAM SAUCE

Does it get any more decadent that roasted chicken thighs bathed in a creamy bacon and mustard sauce? No, and it doesn't get much easier, either! Serve with a simple side salad and a crisp, dry white wine to cut through some of the fat.

YIELD: 4 servings　PREP TIME: 10 minutes　COOK TIME: 30 minutes

8 bone-in, skin-on chicken thighs, about 4 ounces each

2 tablespoons canola oil

½ cup Bacon Mustard Cream Sauce (page 213)

2 teaspoons minced fresh thyme

sea salt

freshly ground pepper

1. Preheat the oven to 400°F. Line a sheet pan with parchment paper.

2. Pat the chicken thighs dry with paper towels. Spread them out on the sheet pan. Brush with the oil and season with salt and pepper. Roast for 25 minutes.

3. During the last 5 minutes of cooking, pour 1 tablespoon of the Bacon Mustard Cream Sauce over each of the chicken thighs and sprinkle with the fresh thyme. Bake for another 5 minutes or until each of the chicken thighs is cooked to an internal temperature of 165°F.

GLUTEN FREE

Nutrition Facts	
(amount per serving)	
Calories	670
Fat	42 g
Protein	66 g
Carbohydrate	2 g
Fiber	0 g

CHICKEN THIGHS WITH MUSHROOMS AND KALE

Mushrooms and kale are flavorful low-carb vegetables that soak up the delicious pan juices of roasted chicken thighs.

YIELD: 4 servings   PREP TIME: 10 minutes   COOK TIME: 30 minutes

8 bone-in, skin-on chicken thighs, about 4 ounces each

3 tablespoons canola oil, divided

2 cups roughly chopped kale

2 cups halved mushrooms

1 teaspoon minced garlic

sea salt

freshly ground pepper

1. Preheat the oven to 400°F. Line a sheet pan with parchment paper.

2. Pat the chicken thighs dry with paper towels. Spread them out on the sheet pan. Brush with 2 tablespoons of the oil and season with salt and pepper. Roast for 15 minutes.

3. Toss the kale and mushrooms with the remaining 1 tablespoon of oil and the garlic. Spread them out on the sheet pan around the par-baked chicken. Season the vegetables with salt and pepper. Bake for another 15 minutes or until the chicken thighs are cooked to an internal temperature of 165°F.

GLUTEN FREE · DAIRY FREE

Nutrition Facts	
(amount per serving)	
Calories	597
Fat	33 g
Protein	65 g
Carbohydrate	5 g
Fiber	1.7 g

MOROCCAN CHICKEN TAGINE

Traditional tagines are prepared in an earthenware vessel with a conical lid to trap steam and slowly cook meat, vegetables, and spices. For those of us without a tagine in our kitchens, a sheet pan covered in foil does the trick. Make sure to use bone-in pieces of chicken to keep it juicy through the long, slow cooking time. Serve with Cauliflower Rice (page 220).

YIELD: 4 servings   PREP TIME: 10 minutes   COOK TIME: 75 minutes

2 yellow onions, sliced in ¼-inch-thick rounds

2 tablespoons olive oil

1 tablespoon curry powder

1 tablespoon ground ginger

1 tablespoon smoked paprika

8 bone-in, skinless chicken thighs

8 cloves garlic, smashed

2 tablespoons roughly chopped preserved lemon

½ cup pitted assorted olives

½ cup chicken broth

sea salt

freshly ground black pepper

½ cup roughly chopped toasted almonds

¼ cup roughly chopped fresh parsley

1. Preheat the oven to 325°F.

2. Spread the onions on a sheet pan and drizzle with the olive oil. Toss gently to coat.

3. In a small bowl, combine the curry powder, ginger, and smoked paprika. Stir in a generous pinch of sea salt and several grinds of black pepper.

4. Coat the chicken thighs in the spice mixture and then set them on top of the onions.

5. Scatter the garlic, preserved lemon, and olives around the chicken. Pour the chicken broth into the pan. Season the whole pan with salt and pepper.

6. Cover the pan tightly with two sheets of aluminum foil.

7. Bake for 1 hour. Remove the foil and continue baking for another 15 minutes. The chicken should be cooked through to an internal temperature of 165°F and the onions will be very soft. Top with almonds and parsley before serving.

GLUTEN FREE · DAIRY FREE · LOW CALORIE

Nutrition Facts	
(amount per serving)	
Calories	356
Fat	21 g
Protein	31 g
Carbohydrate	12 g
Fiber	3 g

BROCCOLI AND CHICKEN SPAGHETTI SQUASH NOODLE BOWL

This is one of my favorite lunch meals after surfing because I'm super hungry and apt to eat a big plate of pasta. This gives me the filling effects without the dreaded carb hangover. Even better, it's super flavorful with a garlic, ginger, and toasted sesame dressing.

YIELD: 4 servings   PREP TIME: 10 minutes   COOK TIME: 30 minutes

1 small spaghetti squash, about 1½ pounds

8 boneless, skinless chicken thighs, cut into 2-inch pieces

2 cups broccoli florets

2 cups halved button mushrooms

1 tablespoon olive oil

1 tablespoon sesame oil

⅓ cup soy sauce

2 tablespoons lime juice

1 teaspoon minced fresh ginger

1 teaspoon minced fresh garlic

sea salt

freshly ground black pepper

1. Preheat the oven to 375°F. Line a sheet pan with parchment paper.

2. Slice the spaghetti squash into 1-inch-thick rings and use a paring knife to remove the seeds and strings. Spread the rings on the sheet pan.

3. In a large bowl, toss the chicken, broccoli, and mushrooms with the olive oil. Season with salt and pepper. Spread the meat and vegetables onto the sheet pan in and around the spaghetti squash.

4. Roast for 30 minutes until the chicken is cooked through and the spaghetti squash is tender.

5. Meanwhile, whisk the sesame oil, soy sauce, lime juice, ginger, and garlic in a small bowl.

6. Remove the pan from the oven and remove the spaghetti squash to a cutting board.

7. Pour the sesame dressing over the chicken and vegetables, tossing gently to coat.

8. Use a fork to shred the spaghetti squash into long, thin strands. Oven mitts are helpful because the squash will still be hot.

9. Divide the spaghetti squash between four serving bowls. Top with the chicken and vegetables, making sure to get some of the sauce.

GLUTEN FREE ▪ DAIRY FREE ▪ LOW CALORIE

Nutrition Facts	
(amount per serving)	
Calories	410
Fat	22 g
Protein	43 g
Carbohydrate	13 g
Fiber	3.5 g

BACON-WRAPPED, GUACAMOLE-STUFFED CHICKEN BREAST

This easy baked chicken breast is stuffed with tangy guacamole and wrapped in smoky bacon. Prepare this at the beginning of the day before you leave for work to make dinner prep a cinch—just pop them in the oven, bake, and enjoy. Add a green vegetable to the pan, such as broccoli or asparagus tossed in olive oil, for a complete meal.

YIELD: 4 servings   PREP TIME: 5 minutes   COOK TIME: 30 minutes

4 boneless, skinless chicken breasts, about 6 ounces each

½ cup Guacamole (page 206)

8 slices applewood-smoked bacon

sea salt

freshly ground black pepper

1. Preheat the oven to 400°F.

2. Pound the chicken breasts to about ¼-inch thickness between two sheets of parchment paper using the flat side of a meat cleaver. Season with salt and pepper.

3. Top each with 2 tablespoons of Guacamole.

4. Roll each of the chicken breasts into a tight cylinder. Wrap each chicken breast in two slices of bacon and secure with a toothpick.

5. Bake for 30 minutes or until the chicken is cooked through and the bacon is beginning to brown.

GLUTEN FREE • DAIRY FREE • LOW CALORIE

Nutrition Facts	
(amount per serving)	
Calories	415
Fat	23 g
Protein	49 g
Carbohydrate	3 g
Fiber	2 g

PESTO CHICKEN AND ASPARAGUS WITH SUN-DRIED TOMATOES

Garlicky pesto and zesty sun-dried tomatoes bring so much flavor to this easy weeknight dinner. You can use the Pesto recipe or a store-bought version. I like to make my own and freeze it in ice cube trays so it is always on hand.

YIELD: 4 servings   PREP TIME: 10 minutes   COOK TIME: 20 minutes

8 boneless, skinless chicken thighs

½ cup Pesto (page 209) or store-bought pesto

1 bunch asparagus, about 1 pound, trimmed

1 tablespoon olive oil

½ cup sliced oil-packed sun-dried tomatoes, drained

sea salt

freshly ground black pepper

1. Preheat the oven to 400°F. Line a sheet pan with parchment paper.

2. Coat the chicken thighs in the Pesto and place them on the sheet pan.

3. Toss the asparagus with the olive oil and season with salt and pepper. Scatter them around the chicken on the sheet pan. Top the asparagus with the sliced sun-dried tomatoes.

4. Bake for 20 minutes or until the chicken is cooked through and the asparagus is soft.

GLUTEN FREE · DAIRY FREE

Nutrition Facts	
(amount per serving)	
Calories	507
Fat	35 g
Protein	43 g
Carbohydrate	10 g
Fiber	4 g

SMOKED GOUDA AND BUTTERNUT SQUASH CHICKEN BAKE

Roasted chicken, onions, and butternut squash are topped with prosciutto and smoked Gouda in this decadent casserole.

YIELD: 4 servings   PREP TIME: 5 minutes   COOK TIME: 30 to 35 minutes

6 boneless, skinless chicken thighs, about 4 ounces each, cut into 2-inch pieces

2 cups cubed butternut squash

1 small onion, halved and sliced into thick rings

1 teaspoon minced fresh rosemary

2 tablespoons coconut oil

4 ounces prosciutto

8 ounces smoked Gouda cheese

sea salt

freshly ground black pepper

1. Preheat the oven to 400°F.

2. Toss the chicken, butternut squash, onion, and rosemary with the coconut oil on a sheet pan. Season with salt and pepper.

3. Roast for 20 minutes until the onions begin to brown and the butternut squash is nearly tender, but not quite.

4. Remove the pan from the oven and top with the prosciutto slices followed by the smoked Gouda.

5. Return the pan to the oven and bake for another 10 to 15 minutes until the cheese is melted and beginning to brown.

GLUTEN FREE

Nutrition Facts	
(amount per serving)	
Calories	557
Fat	33 g
Protein	52 g
Carbohydrate	14 g
Fiber	3.3 g

CHEESY CHICKEN FAJITA BAKE

Roasting the chicken and vegetables briefly first gives them a delicious flavor and ensures that they're thoroughly cooked when the cheese is done. It is meant to be enjoyed as it is, but if you have low-carb wraps, they make an excellent filling.

YIELD: 4 servings   PREP TIME: 5 minutes   COOK TIME: 25 to 30 minutes

8 boneless, skinless chicken thighs, about 4 ounces each

1 small onion, halved and sliced into thick rings

1 green bell pepper, cored and thinly sliced

2 tablespoons canola oil

8 ounces cream cheese

1¾ cups Enchilada Sauce (page 211), or 1 can store-bought

2 cups shredded Mexican blend cheese

sea salt

freshly ground black pepper

1. Preheat the oven to 400°F.

2. Toss the chicken, onion, bell pepper, and oil on the sheet pan. Season with salt and pepper.

3. Roast for 15 minutes until the onions begin to brown.

4. Drop the cream cheese by the spoonful over and around the chicken and peppers. Pour the Enchilada Sauce over the pan, trying to disperse it all over. Top with the shredded cheese.

5. Return the pan to the oven and bake for another 10 to 15 minutes until the cheese is bubbling and beginning to brown. Allow to rest for 5 minutes before serving.

GLUTEN FREE

Nutrition Facts	
(amount per serving)	
Calories	689
Fat	52 g
Protein	46 g
Carbohydrate	11 g
Fiber	1.4 g

CHICKEN AND HERB-ROASTED VEGETABLES

These roasted vegetables flavored with fresh thyme and rosemary are a delicious backdrop to roasted chicken thighs. Although the total carbs are on the upper end, there are only 10 grams of net carbs per serving.

YIELD: 4 servings   PREP TIME: 10 minutes   COOK TIME: 35 minutes

3 zucchini, cut into 1-inch pieces

1 red onion, halved and sliced in ¼-inch slices

1 medium beet, peeled and quartered

2 carrots, unpeeled, cut into 2-inch pieces

1 tablespoon minced fresh thyme

1 teaspoon minced fresh rosemary

2 tablespoons olive oil

8 bone-in, skin-on chicken thighs, about 4 ounces each

1 teaspoon red wine vinegar

sea salt

freshly ground pepper

1. Preheat the oven to 375°F. Line a sheet pan with parchment paper.

2. Spread the zucchini, onion, beet, and carrots onto the sheet pan. Season with thyme and rosemary. Drizzle with olive oil and toss gently to coat.

3. Add the chicken thighs to the pan around the vegetables. Season with salt and pepper.

4. Roast uncovered for 35 minutes or until the chicken is cooked through to an internal temperature of 165°F.

5. Remove the chicken thighs to a serving dish. Toss the vegetables with red wine vinegar and serve alongside the chicken.

GLUTEN FREE · DAIRY FREE

Nutrition Facts	
(amount per serving)	
Calories	554
Fat	32 g
Protein	52 g
Carbohydrate	14 g
Fiber	4 g

ROASTED CHICKEN LEG QUARTERS WITH BACON AND BRUSSELS SPROUTS

Smoky bacon permeates the Brussels sprouts in this rich, filling entree. If you cannot find full chicken legs, swap them for eight bone-in chicken thighs.

YIELD: 4 servings   PREP TIME: 5 minutes   COOK TIME: 40 minutes

4 bone-in, skin-on chicken leg quarters (legs and thighs)

2 tablespoons rendered bacon fat or coconut oil, divided

1 medium yellow onion, halved and sliced in quarter-inch-thick slices

4 cups halved Brussels sprouts

4 slices thick-cut bacon, sliced into ½-inch pieces

sea salt

freshly ground pepper

1. Preheat the oven to 400°F.

2. Coat the chicken pieces with 1 tablespoon of the rendered bacon fat and season with salt and pepper. Place on the sheet pan and roast for 20 minutes.

3. Toss the onion, Brussels sprouts, and bacon pieces in the remaining bacon fat. Season with salt and pepper.

4. Spread them on the sheet pan and roast for another 20 minutes or until the vegetables are soft and the chicken is cooked through to an internal temperature of 165°F.

GLUTEN FREE • DAIRY FREE

Nutrition Facts	
(amount per serving)	
Calories	509
Fat	32 g
Protein	43 g
Carbohydrate	10 g
Fiber	3.8 g

BASIC ROASTED CHICKEN

Learning how to roast a whole chicken rather than purchasing pre-butchered parts slashed my grocery bill for meat and yielded much more flavorful chicken dinners. I have used both a sheet pan and a traditional roasting pan for chicken, but the sheet pan works better to get the skin nice and crispy. Use oil instead of butter to make this chicken dairy free.

YIELD: 4 servings   PREP TIME: 10 minutes   COOK TIME: 40 minutes

1 whole chicken, with skin, about 3 to 4 pounds

1 clove garlic, halved

2 tablespoons oil or butter

1 tablespoon minced fresh herbs (optional)

1 teaspoon lemon zest (optional)

sea salt

freshly ground pepper

1. Preheat the oven to 450°F.

2. Using a serrated knife or sharp kitchen shears, cut down one side of the chicken backbone, slicing through the ribs. Carefully cut down the other side to remove the backbone. Reserve it for another use, such as making stock.

3. Season the open cavity of the chicken with salt and pepper. Place the chicken onto the sheet pan with the cut-side down, spreading out the legs. Press down between the breasts to flatten the chicken. Pat it dry with paper towels.

4. Rub the chicken all over with the cut side of the garlic, then coat in the oil or butter. Season with salt, pepper, herbs, and lemon zest (if using).

5. Bake for 10 minutes, then reduce the heat to 325°F.

6. Bake for another 30 minutes or until the chicken is cooked through and reaches an internal temperature of 155°F. It will continue cooking after it comes out of the oven and reach an internal temperature of 165°F. Allow the chicken to rest for 10 minutes before slicing and serving.

GLUTEN FREE ▪ DAIRY FREE ▪ LOW CALORIE

Nutrition Facts
(amount per serving)

Calories	454
Fat	34 g
Protein	34 g
Carbohydrate	0 g
Fiber	0 g

SMOKY GARLIC BUTTER WHOLE ROASTED CHICKEN AND SPINACH

The flavors of chipotle, smoked paprika, and garlic infuse the chicken with flavor. Butter and an initial blast of heat gets the skin deliciously crispy. Serve with Mashed Cauliflower (page 221).

YIELD: 4 servings   PREP TIME: 10 minutes   COOK TIME: 40 minutes

1 whole chicken, with skin, about 3 to 4 pounds

½ stick (½ cup) Smoky Garlic Compound Butter (page 201), softened

1 bunch spinach, stems discarded, roughly chopped

sea salt

freshly ground pepper

1. Preheat the oven to 450°F.

2. Using a serrated knife or sharp kitchen shears, cut down one side of the chicken backbone, slicing through the ribs. Carefully cut down the other side to remove the backbone. Reserve it for another use, such as making stock.

3. Season the open cavity of the chicken with salt and pepper. Place the chicken onto the sheet pan with the cut-side down, spreading out the legs. Press down between the breasts to flatten the chicken. Pat it dry with paper towels.

4. Rub the compound butter all over the chicken, reaching underneath the skin.

5. Bake for 10 minutes, then reduce the heat to 325°F.

6. Bake for another 30 minutes or until the chicken is cooked through and reaches an internal temperature of 155°F. It will continue cooking after it comes out of the oven and reach an internal temperature of 165°F.

7. During the last 3 minutes of cooking, add the spinach to the pan and toss it in the pan juices and fat. Return to the oven and cook just until wilted.

8. Allow the chicken to rest for 10 minutes before slicing and serving.

GLUTEN FREE • LOW CALORIE

Nutrition Facts	
(amount per serving)	
Calories	466
Fat	34 g
Protein	34 g
Carbohydrate	3 g
Fiber	1.9 g

WHOLE ROASTED CHICKEN WITH ZUCCHINI, ONIONS, AND CARROTS

This is one of my go-to recipes for roasted chicken and vegetables. All of the juices from the chicken spill out onto the pan, flavoring the zucchini and onions.

YIELD: 4 servings   PREP TIME: 10 minutes   COOK TIME: 35 to 40 minutes

1 whole chicken, with skin, about 3 to 4 pounds

2 tablespoons Garlic Herb Compound Butter (page 200)

2 cups diced zucchini

1 small red onion, thinly sliced

2 medium carrots, unpeeled, halved and cut into 1-inch pieces

1 tablespoon canola oil

sea salt

freshly ground pepper

1. Preheat the oven to 425°F.

2. Using a serrated knife or sharp kitchen shears, cut down one side of the chicken backbone, slicing through the ribs. Carefully cut down the other side to remove the backbone. Reserve it for another use, such as making stock.

3. Season the open cavity of the chicken with salt and pepper. Place the chicken onto the sheet pan with the cut-side down, spreading out the legs. Press down between the breasts to flatten the chicken. Pat it dry with paper towels.

4. Rub the compound butter all over the chicken, reaching underneath the skin.

5. Bake for 15 minutes, then reduce the heat to 325°F. Add the vegetables to the pan and toss them in the pan juices and canola oil.

6. Bake for another 20 to 25 minutes or until the chicken is cooked through and reaches an internal temperature of 155°F and the vegetables are soft and beginning to brown. The chicken will continue cooking after it comes out of the oven and reach an internal temperature of 165°F.

7. Allow the chicken to rest for 10 minutes before slicing and serving.

GLUTEN FREE ▪ LOW CALORIE

Nutrition Facts	
(amount per serving)	
Calories	517
Fat	34 g
Protein	39 g
Carbohydrate	8 g
Fiber	2.4 g

SAUSAGE, FENNEL, AND CHICKEN DRUMSTICKS

This recipe appears in my book Sheet Pan Paleo, *but the caramelized fennel, spicy Italian sausage, and juicy chicken drumsticks are so delicious—and naturally low-carb—I wanted to include it here as well. If you're making this for younger palates, consider opting for mild Italian sausage.*

YIELD: 4 servings   PREP TIME: 5 minutes   COOK TIME: 40 to 45 minutes

2 fennel bulbs, sliced into 8 wedges

4 hot Italian sausages, sliced into 1-inch pieces

8 chicken drumsticks

¼ cup olive oil

sea salt

freshly ground pepper

1. Preheat the oven to 375°F. Line a sheet pan with parchment paper.

2. Arrange the fennel, sausage, and chicken drumsticks on the sheet pan. Drizzle with the olive oil and toss gently to coat. Season with salt and pepper.

3. Bake for 40 to 45 minutes or until the chicken is cooked through to an internal temperature of 165°F and the fennel is soft.

GLUTEN FREE • DAIRY FREE • LOW CALORIE

Nutrition Facts	
(amount per serving)	
Calories	613
Fat	46 g
Protein	39 g
Carbohydrate	9 g
Fiber	3.7 g

CHAPTER SEVEN

Pork

The ketogenic diet makes a fantastic excuse to indulge in the forbidden food among low-fat dieters—bacon! This chapter is filled with plenty of everyone's favorite indulgence, along with ground pork, pork tenderloin, and the best barbecue ribs you may ever have.

PORK MARSALA

Pork Marsala is the epitome of comfort food—the earthy mushrooms, heady Marsala wine, and aromatic herbs, garlic, and onions all enliven the tender pork loin chops. It gets even better with cold butter whisked into the Marsala to form a luxurious pan sauce. This is a complete meal on its own, or serve with Mashed Cauliflower (page 221) for a decadent dinner.

YIELD: 4 servings   PREP TIME: 10 minutes   COOK TIME: 20 minutes

3 cups halved cremini or button mushrooms

1 medium yellow onion, halved and thinly sliced

2 cloves garlic, minced

1 teaspoon minced fresh rosemary

4 boneless pork loin chops, about 6 ounces each

4 tablespoons canola oil, divided

1 tablespoon coconut flour

1 teaspoon garlic powder

½ teaspoon onion powder

½ teaspoon sea salt

½ teaspoon freshly ground pepper

½ cup Marsala wine

2 tablespoons cold butter

1. Preheat the oven to 400°F.

2. Toss the mushrooms, onion, and garlic with 2 tablespoons of the canola oil on the sheet pan. Season with salt and pepper.

3. Pound the pork loin chops with a meat mallet until they are about ½ inch thick. Pat the chops dry with paper towels and then coat in 2 tablespoons of the canola oil.

4. Combine the coconut flour, garlic powder, onion powder, salt, and pepper in a small bowl. Lightly coat the pork chops in the flour mixture and lay them on the sheet pan, pushing the vegetables aside as needed so the meat makes full contact with the pan.

5. Roast for 10 minutes. Remove the pan from the oven and flip the pork chops.

6. Add the Marsala wine to the pan and cook for another 5 to 7 minutes until the pork is cooked to a temperature of 145°F.

7. Transfer the pork and vegetables to individual serving plates, leaving the Marsala in the pan.

8. Whisk the cold butter into the Marsala until it thickens slightly. Carefully spoon the sauce over the pork and mushrooms.

GLUTEN FREE · LOW CALORIE

Nutrition Facts	
(amount per serving)	
Calories	351
Fat	19 g
Protein	35 g
Carbohydrate	8 g
Fiber	2.2 g

PROSCIUTTO AND GOUDA-STUFFED PORK

I'll admit, this recipe is a little over the top. Creamy smoked Gouda cheese, salty prosciutto, and fragrant minced rosemary fill each pork loin chop, which is then coated in olive oil and breaded in grated Parmesan. As in other instances in this book where Parmesan is used for breading, the canned grated Parmesan really is your best bet. This dish is a perfect balance of flavors and textures, but if you want to serve it with Bacon Mustard Cream Sauce (page 213), go for it!

YIELD: 4 servings   PREP TIME: 10 minutes   COOK TIME: 20 to 25 minutes

4 pork loin chops, about 6 ounces each

1 tablespoon minced rosemary

4 slices prosciutto

4 ounces sliced smoked Gouda cheese

2 tablespoons olive oil

½ cup grated Parmesan cheese

sea salt

freshly ground pepper

1. Preheat the oven to 400°F. Line a sheet pan with parchment paper.

2. Pound the pork loin with a meat mallet to about ⅛ to ¼ inch thickness. Season it liberally with salt, pepper, and rosemary.

3. Lay a slice of prosciutto over each piece of meat. Top with 1 slice of the smoked Gouda.

4. Roll the pork into a tight cylinder and secure with a toothpick. Repeat with the remaining chops and filling ingredients.

5. Rub the pork rolls with the olive oil and then coat with the Parmesan cheese.

6. Bake for 20 to 25 minutes until the pork is cooked through and the cheese is oozing out.

GLUTEN FREE • LOW CALORIE

Nutrition Facts
(amount per serving)

Calories	496
Fat	33 g
Protein	47 g
Carbohydrate	3 g
Fiber	0 g

SLOW-ROASTED BARBECUE RIBS

I usually make ribs on the grill, but even in Southern California, summer eventually ends and I take my cooking back inside. That turned out to be the best thing that ever happened to this recipe. You'll see what I mean when you make it. The long, slow roast in the oven produces tender meat that falls off the bone before it is saturated with a rich, flavorful barbecue sauce. Plus, no risk of flare-ups on the grill!

YIELD: 6 servings   PREP TIME: 10 minutes, plus minimum 30 minutes inactive time   COOK TIME: 2 hours 45 minutes

For the brine:

¼ cup sea salt

7 cups water

1 bay leaf

1 teaspoon whole peppercorns

4 cups ice

For the ribs:

1 rack pork ribs, 2 to 3 pounds, halved

1 tablespoon canola oil

1 teaspoon smoked paprika

½ teaspoon ground cumin

½ teaspoon onion powder

½ teaspoon garlic powder (not salt)

For the sauce:

¾ cup Barbecue Sauce (page 212)

¼ cup roughly chopped cilantro

1 scallion, white and green parts

1. To make the brine, dissolve the salt into 1 cup of boiling water. Add 1 bay leaf and a teaspoon of peppercorns. Cool the mixture with 6 additional cups of ice water.

2. Place the ribs into a glass baking dish, meat-side down. Pour the brine over the ribs and place the dish into the refrigerator on the bottom shelf. Cover and brine for at least 30 minutes and up to 8 hours.

3. To cook the ribs, preheat the oven to 250°F.

4. Remove the ribs from the brine and pat dry with paper towels. Coat with the canola oil.

5. Combine the paprika, cumin, onion powder, and garlic powder in a small bowl. Rub this over the meat.

6. Place the ribs meat-side down on a sheet pan. Cover the pan tightly with foil. Bake for 2½ hours.

7. Remove the pan from the oven and remove the foil. Carefully transfer the ribs to a separate dish.

8. Pour ½ cup of the cooking liquid into a blender and discard the rest. Add the Barbecue Sauce, cilantro, and scallion to the blender and puree until smooth.

9. Return the ribs to the sheet pan and pour half of the Barbecue Sauce over them. Return to the oven and roast for another 15 minutes. Serve the remaining sauce on the side.

GLUTEN FREE · DAIRY FREE

Nutrition Facts (amount per serving)	
Calories	736
Fat	58 g
Protein	46 g
Carbohydrate	4 g
Fiber	0.3 g

CITRUS AND HERB MARINATED PORK SHOULDER

Cuban flavors permeate this slow-roasted pork shoulder. It serves eight but is also perfect for meal prep at the beginning of the week. Serve it with Savoy Cabbage and Almond Slaw (page 217) for a filling meal.

YIELD: 8 servings   PREP TIME: 10 minutes, plus 8 hours inactive time
COOK TIME: 2 to 2½ hours

½ cup olive oil

zest and juice of 1 orange

zest and juice of 1 lime

1 cup minced fresh cilantro

¼ cup minced fresh mint leaves

8 cloves garlic, minced

2 teaspoons ground cumin

1 teaspoon ground coriander

3- to 4-pound bone-in pork shoulder

sea salt

freshly ground pepper

1. Combine the oil, citrus juices and zest, herbs, garlic, and spices in a zip-top bag. Season with 1 teaspoon each of salt and pepper. Place the pork shoulder in the marinade and turn to coat thoroughly. Cover and refrigerate overnight.

2. To cook the pork, preheat the oven to 450°F. Place an oven-safe baking rack over the sheet pan.

3. Remove the pork shoulder from the marinade and set it on the rack. Season generously with salt and pepper. Roast uncovered for 30 minutes, then reduce the oven temperature to 325°F and cook for another 1½ to 2 hours or until the pork is cooked to an internal temperature of 160°F.

4. Remove to a cutting board to rest for 15 to 20 minutes before slicing.

GLUTEN FREE ▪ DAIRY FREE

Nutrition Facts	
(amount per serving)	
Calories	671
Fat	54 g
Protein	41 g
Carbohydrate	3 g
Fiber	0.5 g

RAINBOW PEPPERCORN PORK CHOPS WITH ENDIVE

The complexity of white, green, pink, and black peppercorns flavors the brine that keeps the pork chops exceptionally juicy while roasting. Endive is a small, bitter, leafed vegetable that is lower in carbs than almost any other vegetable, including asparagus. It provides a lovely contrast in texture and flavor to the pork chops.

YIELD: 4 servings   PREP TIME: 10 minutes, plus minimum 1 hour inactive time   COOK TIME: 20 minutes

1 cup water	4 bone-in pork chops, about 6 to 8 ounces each
¼ cup multicolored peppercorns	2 heads endive, halved lengthwise
1 tablespoon sea salt	zest and juice of 1 lemon
3 cloves garlic, minced, divided	4 tablespoons olive oil, divided
2 tablespoons red wine vinegar	sea salt
2 cups ice	freshly ground pepper

1. Bring the water to a simmer in a saucepan with the peppercorns, sea salt, and 1 clove garlic, stirring until the salt is dissolved. Stir in the red wine vinegar. Cool the mixture by adding 2 cups of ice.

2. Place the pork chops in a non-reactive dish and pour the cooled brine over and around. Place in the refrigerator for at least 1 hour and cover and brine up to 8 hours.

3. To cook the pork, preheat the oven to 400°F. Line a sheet pan with parchment paper.

4. Coat the endive in the remaining garlic cloves, lemon zest, and 3 tablespoons of the olive oil. Season with salt and pepper. Spread the endive on the sheet pan.

5. Remove the pork from the brine and pat dry with paper towels. Coat with the remaining olive oil and season generously with pepper. Place alongside the endive.

6. Roast uncovered for 20 minutes or until the chops register an internal temperature between 140 and 145°F.

7. Shower the endive with the lemon juice just before serving.

GLUTEN FREE ▪ DAIRY FREE

Nutrition Facts	
(amount per serving)	
Calories	380
Fat	24 g
Protein	35 g
Carbohydrate	10 g
Fiber	9.5 g

PORK TENDERLOIN WITH RADISHES AND OLIVE MAYO

Juicy and delicious pork tenderloin gets upstaged by the tender roasted radishes and briny olive aioli in this complete one-pan dinner.

YIELD: 4 servings   PREP TIME: 10 minutes   COOK TIME: 20 minutes

1 pound pork tenderloin

3 tablespoons olive oil, divided

2 bunches radishes, thoroughly washed

juice of 1 lemon

½ cup mayonnaise

4 Kalamata olives, minced

1 clove garlic, minced

sea salt

freshly ground pepper

1. Preheat the oven to 450°F. Line a sheet pan with parchment paper.

2. Pat the pork loin dry with paper towels. Coat with 1 tablespoon of the oil and season with salt and pepper. Place it on the center of the sheet pan.

3. Cut the tops off the radishes and set the greens aside, leaving about 1 inch of the stem. Halve the radishes lengthwise and toss with an additional 2 tablespoons of oil. Place them cut-side down on the sheet pan. Season with salt and pepper.

4. Roast uncovered for 20 minutes or until the pork loin registers an internal temperature between 140 and 145°F. Remove the pork to a cutting board and cover with foil for 10 minutes before slicing.

5. While the pork is resting, make the sauce by whisking the lemon juice, mayonnaise, olives, and garlic together in a small bowl.

6. Check the radish greens for any grit or wilted leaves and then slice into thin ribbons. Toss them with the roasted radishes on the sheet pan.

7. To serve, divide the sliced pork between plates. Serve the radishes, greens, and the olive mayonnaise on the side.

GLUTEN FREE ▪ DAIRY FREE

Nutrition Facts	
(amount per serving)	
Calories	543
Fat	44 g
Protein	34 g
Carbohydrate	3 g
Fiber	0.7 g

SMOKY PORK TENDERLOIN WITH CRISPY CABBAGE

This pork tenderloin is coated in a piquant, savory spice rub. It makes excellent leftovers and is delicious served with Cauliflower Rice (page 220).

YIELD: 4 servings   PREP TIME: 10 minutes   COOK TIME: 20 minutes

1 tablespoon smoked paprika

1 teaspoon ground chipotle

1 teaspoon ground cumin

½ teaspoon garlic powder

½ teaspoon onion powder

1 teaspoon sea salt

½ teaspoon freshly ground pepper

1 pound pork tenderloin

2 tablespoons canola oil

4 cups shredded red cabbage

1. Preheat the oven to 450°F. Line a sheet pan with parchment paper.

2. Combine the paprika, chipotle, cumin, garlic powder, onion powder, salt, and pepper in a small bowl. Reserve 1 teaspoon of this mixture for the cabbage.

3. Pat the meat dry with paper towels. Coat with 1 tablespoon of the oil and season with the spice rub. Place it on the center of the sheet pan.

4. Toss the cabbage with the remaining tablespoon of oil and the remaining teaspoon of the spice rub. Spread it around the pork on the sheet pan.

5. Roast the pork uncovered for 20 minutes or until the pork loin registers an internal temperature between 140 and 145°F. Remove the pork to a cutting board and cover with foil for 10 minutes before slicing.

GLUTEN FREE ▪ DAIRY FREE ▪ LOW CALORIE

Nutrition Facts	
(amount per serving)	
Calories	338
Fat	18 g
Protein	37 g
Carbohydrate	6 g
Fiber	2.7 g

ITALIAN MEATBALLS

Herbs and garlic permeate these juicy meatballs. The fennel seed gives this an Italian sausage vibe, but if you don't have it in your pantry, feel free to omit it. The meatballs are delicious served on their own or with a low-carb marinara sauce and spiralized zucchini.

YIELD: 6 servings   PREP TIME: 10 minutes   COOK TIME: 25 minutes

1 pound ground pork

1 pound ground beef

1 cup grated onions

1 tablespoon minced garlic

1 tablespoon Italian herb blend

1 teaspoon ground fennel seed (optional)

1½ teaspoons sea salt

½ teaspoon freshly ground pepper

1 egg, whisked

1 cup grated Parmesan cheese

½ cup diced plum tomatoes

1. Preheat the oven to 400°F. Line a sheet pan with parchment paper.

2. Combine the pork, beef, onions, garlic, Italian herb blend, fennel (if using), sea salt, pepper, egg, and Parmesan in a large bowl. Do not overmix. Fold in the plum tomatoes.

3. Form the mixture into 12 large meatballs, about 2 to 3 inches in diameter, and place them onto the sheet pan. Bake for 25 minutes or until just cooked through. Do not overcook or they will get tough.

GLUTEN FREE

Nutrition Facts	
(amount per serving)	
Calories	563
Fat	42 g
Protein	41 g
Carbohydrate	4 g
Fiber	0.8 g

HAM IN TOMATO CREAM SAUCE

This French-style baked ham in a velvety tomato cream sauce is adapted from a recipe for Jambon Au Chablis in Saveur *magazine. My version cuts the cooking time and the carbs in half, but it's still rich and delicious.*

YIELD: 4 servings   PREP TIME: 5 minutes   COOK TIME: 25 to 30 minutes

1 pound cooked ham, sliced ¼-inch thick

½ cup chicken stock

1 tablespoon white wine vinegar

2 tablespoons tomato paste

1 shallot, minced

1 tablespoon minced fresh tarragon

2 cups heavy cream

sea salt

freshly ground pepper

1. Preheat the oven to 400°F.

2. Spread the ham slices out on the sheet pan.

3. Combine the chicken stock, vinegar, tomato paste, shallot, and tarragon in a blender. Puree until smooth. Add the heavy cream and pulse a few times, just until integrated. Season to taste with salt and pepper.

4. Pour the cream sauce over the ham, turning each slice to coat thoroughly. Bake uncovered for 25 to 30 minutes until the sauce is bubbling and the ham is gently browned.

GLUTEN FREE

Nutrition Facts	
(amount per serving)	
Calories	678
Fat	58 g
Protein	26 g
Carbohydrate	13 g
Fiber	1 g

VIETNAMESE PORK MEATBALL LETTUCE WRAPS

These scrumptious lettuce wraps make a tasty appetizer for four or a filling dinner for two.

YIELD: 4 servings   PREP TIME: 10 minutes   COOK TIME: 15 to 17 minutes

1 pound ground pork

1 tablespoon minced ginger

1 teaspoon minced garlic

2 scallions, white and green parts, thinly sliced on a bias, divided

½ cup roughly chopped cilantro, divided

1 tablespoon fish sauce

½ cup shredded carrot

1 cup shredded cabbage

juice of 1 lime

½ cup roughly chopped dry-roasted peanuts

1 head butter lettuce

1. Preheat the oven to 400°F. Line a sheet pan with parchment paper.

2. Combine the pork, ginger, garlic, half of the scallions, half of the cilantro, and the fish sauce in a medium bowl. Form into 12 meatballs and place them on the sheet pan.

3. Bake uncovered for 10 minutes, then turn over and continue baking for another 5 to 7 minutes or until the pork is cooked through.

4. While the meatballs are baking, combine the remaining scallion, cilantro, carrot, and cabbage in a medium bowl. Squeeze the lime juice over the top.

5. To serve, place three meatballs in a lettuce leaf along with a pinch of shredded carrot mixture. Top with the peanuts.

GLUTEN FREE ▪ DAIRY FREE ▪ LOW CALORIE

Nutrition Facts
(amount per serving)

Calories	469
Fat	33 g
Protein	35 g
Carbohydrate	9 g
Fiber	3.2 g

HAWAIIAN PIZZA WITH CAULIFLOWER CRUST

Who says a low-carb diet can't include fruit? Judicious use of diced pineapple brightens the appearance and flavor of this loaded pizza. I am not sure how Canadian bacon and pineapple came to represent Hawaiian pizza, but it sure tastes good!

YIELD: 4 servings   PREP TIME: 15 minutes   COOK TIME: 18 to 20 minutes

1 medium head cauliflower, broken into florets

½ teaspoon sea salt

1 egg

½ cup grated Parmesan cheese

¼ cup almond flour

½ cup Marinara Sauce (page 210) or store-bought, no-sugar-added marinara

16 ounces shredded mozzarella

4 ounces Canadian bacon

½ cup diced pineapple, fresh or canned without added sugar

1. Preheat the oven to 425°F. Line a sheet pan with parchment paper.

2. Using the grater attachment on your food processor, grate the cauliflower. If you do not have a food processor, you can use a box grater, but it will take a while.

3. To prepare the cauliflower, spread it in a microwave-safe baking dish and microwave on high for 3 minutes. Stir and microwave again for 2 minutes. Set aside to cool for 10 minutes.

4. When the cauliflower is cool enough to handle, use your hands to squeeze as much of the moisture out of it as you can.

5. Thoroughly mix the cauliflower with the sea salt, egg, Parmesan cheese, and almond flour.

6. Press the mixture into the sheet pan in a circle, or spread it all the way to the edges for a thinner crust.

7. Bake for 12 minutes until the crust is beginning to brown.

8. Brush the top of the crust with Marinara Sauce and top with the mozzarella, Canadian bacon, and pineapple. Bake for another 8 to 10 minutes or until the mozzarella is melted and beginning to brown.

GLUTEN FREE

Nutrition Facts	
(amount per serving)	
Calories	554
Fat	36 g
Protein	42 g
Carbohydrate	17 g
Fiber	4.8 g

SAUSAGE PIZZA WITH CAULIFLOWER CRUST

This pizza is a meat-lover's dream. It is loaded with Italian sausage and pepperoni, along with melty fontina cheese and fragrant rosemary. If you cannot find precooked Italian sausage, purchase the uncooked links and brown in a skillet for 5 to 10 minutes, or until fully cooked, before adding to the pizza.

YIELD: 4 servings   PREP TIME: 15 minutes   COOK TIME: 20 to 30 minutes

1 medium head cauliflower, broken into florets

½ teaspoon sea salt

1 egg

½ cup grated Parmesan cheese

¼ cup almond flour

½ cup Marinara Sauce (page 210) or store-bought, no-sugar-added marinara

8 ounces fontina cheese, sliced

8 ounces crumbled precooked Italian sausage

4 ounces pepperoni

½ small red onion, thinly sliced

1 teaspoon minced fresh rosemary

1. Preheat the oven to 425°F. Line a sheet pan with parchment paper.

2. Using the grater attachment on your food processor, grate the cauliflower. If you do not have a food processor, you can use a box grater, but it will take a while.

3. To prepare the cauliflower, spread it in a microwave-safe baking dish and microwave on high for 3 minutes. Stir and microwave again for 2 minutes. Set aside to cool for 10 minutes.

4. When the cauliflower is cool enough to handle, use your hands to squeeze as much of the moisture out of it as you can.

5. Thoroughly mix the cauliflower with the sea salt, egg, Parmesan cheese, and almond flour.

6. Press the mixture into the sheet pan in a circle, or spread it all the way to the edges for a thinner crust.

7. Bake for 12 minutes until the crust is beginning to brown.

8. Brush the top of the crust with marinara sauce and top with the fontina, Italian sausage, pepperoni, onion, and rosemary. Bake for another 8 to 10 minutes or until the fontina is melted and beginning to brown.

GLUTEN FREE

Nutrition Facts	
(amount per serving)	
Calories	660
Fat	50 g
Protein	40 g
Carbohydrate	14.5 g
Fiber	5.2 g

BROCCOLI, HAM, AND MOZZARELLA BAKE

If you're craving a rich, cheesy casserole, try this Broccoli, Ham, and Mozzarella Bake. It's simple and delicious and packs a few grams of fiber into each serving. I'm not normally a fan of frozen vegetables, but they really work here.

YIELD: 4 servings   PREP TIME: 5 minutes   COOK TIME: 20 minutes

16 ounces frozen broccoli, defrosted

16 ounces ham, cut into ½-inch pieces

2 cloves garlic, minced

2 tablespoons canola oil

16 ounces fresh mozzarella, sliced

sea salt

freshly ground pepper

1. Preheat the oven to 375°F. Line a sheet pan with parchment paper.

2. Toss the broccoli, ham, garlic, and canola oil on the sheet pan. Season with salt and pepper.

3. Spread the sliced mozzarella over the broccoli and ham.

4. Bake for 20 minutes until the cheese is browned and bubbling.

GLUTEN FREE

Nutrition Facts	
(amount per serving)	
Calories	660
Fat	46 g
Protein	51 g
Carbohydrate	12 g
Fiber	3.4 g

CHAPTER EIGHT

Beef and Lamb

When people think of low-carb diets, endless lettuce-wrapped burgers are one of the first things to come to mind. Fortunately, there's so much more to ketogenic cooking than burgers! In this chapter, I explore some of the more decadent cuts of steak and include the ever-flavorful ground beef along with bison and lamb. I draw from cuisines around the globe for fresh, interesting meals created around these mainstay meats.

FLATIRON STEAKS WITH CREAMED SPINACH

Creamy spiced spinach serves as the perfect backdrop for slices of tender flatiron steak.

YIELD: 4 servings   PREP TIME: 5 minutes   COOK TIME: 12 to 15 minutes

16-ounce flatiron steak

2 tablespoons olive oil, divided

1 pound fresh spinach

2 cloves garlic, minced

1 teaspoon lemon zest

1/8 teaspoon grated nutmeg

1/3 cup heavy cream, warmed

sea salt

freshly ground pepper

1. Preheat the oven to 400°F. Line a sheet pan with parchment paper.

2. Coat the steak with 1 tablespoon of the olive oil. Season liberally with salt and pepper.

3. Roast for 7 minutes.

4. In a small bowl, combine the remaining tablespoon olive oil, spinach, garlic, lemon zest, and nutmeg. Season with salt and pepper.

5. Remove the steak from the oven and flip the steak. Spread the spinach mixture around the steak. Roast for another 5 to 8 minutes or until the spinach is soft and the steak is cooked through but soft.

6. Allow the steak to rest for 5 minutes before slicing.

7. Transfer the spinach to a blender or food processor and add the cream. Pulse a few times until creamy but still slightly chunky. Adjust seasoning with salt and pepper. Serve the spinach alongside the steak.

GLUTEN FREE · LOW CALORIE

Nutrition Facts	
(amount per serving)	
Calories	343
Fat	24 g
Protein	27 g
Carbohydrate	6 g
Fiber	2.8 g

BACON-WRAPPED FILET MIGNON

Filet mignon is so tender and flavorful, it needs little accompaniment to make it shine. Then again, everything is better with bacon, so pick an applewood-smoked variety or another thick-cut bacon.

YIELD: 4 servings   PREP TIME: 5 minutes   COOK TIME: 15 minutes

4 filet mignon steaks, 4 to 6 ounces each

4 slices thick-cut bacon

1 tablespoons olive oil

sea salt

freshly ground pepper

1. Preheat the oven to 425°F.

2. Wrap 1 slice of bacon around each of the filets, securing with a toothpick.

3. Rub the top and bottom of the steaks with the olive oil and season with salt and pepper.

4. Place the filets on the sheet pan and roast for 15 minutes for medium-rare or until they reach your desired level of doneness.

GLUTEN FREE ▪ DAIRY FREE ▪ LOW CALORIE

Nutrition Facts	
(amount per serving)	
Calories	450
Fat	34 g
Protein	31 g
Carbohydrate	0 g
Fiber	0 g

CHINESE BEEF AND BROCCOLI

Skip the carb-heavy takeout in favor of this easy Chinese restaurant standby.

YIELD: 2 servings   PREP TIME: 10 minutes   COOK TIME: 20 minutes

1 small head broccoli, cut into small florets

1 tablespoon toasted sesame oil

1 tablespoon minced garlic

½ teaspoon red chile flakes

1 tablespoon soy sauce

2 boneless rib eye steaks, about 8 ounces each

1 tablespoon canola oil

juice of 1 lime

sea salt

freshly ground pepper

1. Preheat the oven to 450°F. Line a sheet pan with parchment paper.

2. Spread the broccoli out on the sheet pan and toss with the sesame oil, garlic, red chile flakes, and soy sauce.

3. Coat the steak with the canola oil and season with salt and pepper. Set it on the sheet pan, making space between the broccoli.

4. Roast for 10 minutes, then lower the temperature to 325°F and cook until the steak reaches an internal temperature of 135 to 140°F, about 10 minutes more.

5. Allow the meat to rest for 10 minutes before slicing very thinly. Toss with the broccoli and season with the lime juice.

GLUTEN FREE • DAIRY FREE

Nutrition Facts	
(amount per serving)	
Calories	610
Fat	51 g
Protein	38 g
Carbohydrate	4 g
Fiber	1.2 g

COFFEE-CRUSTED RIB EYE STEAK

Bone-in rib eye steaks are incredibly flavorful and offer a generous ratio of fat to protein. The coffee, herb, and garlic rub infuses the steaks with flavor, especially if you can allow them to rest for several hours in the rub before cooking.

YIELD: 4 servings   PREP TIME: 30 minutes   COOK TIME: 15 minutes

2 tablespoons ground coffee

1 tablespoon minced fresh rosemary

1 teaspoon sea salt

1 teaspoon garlic powder

1 teaspoon onion powder

½ teaspoon red chile flakes

4 bone-in rib eye steaks, about 8 to 10 ounces each

1 tablespoon olive oil

freshly ground pepper

1. Preheat the oven to 500°F. Line a sheet pan with foil to make cleanup easier.

2. Combine the coffee, rosemary, sea salt, garlic powder, onion powder, and red chile flakes in a small bowl.

3. Pat the steaks dry with paper towels and then coat with the olive oil. Press the coffee rub into the meat and leave out at room temperature for at least 30 minutes. If you have extra time, wrap the steaks in plastic wrap and set in the refrigerator for several hours to allow the flavors to permeate the meat.

4. Set an oven-safe baking rack over the sheet pan and set the steaks on the rack. Roast for 5 minutes.

5. Reduce the heat to 325°F and continue roasting for another 10 minutes or until the meat reaches an internal temperature of 145°F. It will continue cooking after coming out of the oven.

6. Allow the meat to rest for 10 minutes before serving.

GLUTEN FREE ▪ DAIRY FREE

Nutrition Facts	
(amount per serving)	
Calories	877
Fat	69 g
Protein	69 g
Carbohydrate	1 g
Fiber	0.2 g

RIB EYE STEAKS WITH ROMESCO AND ROASTED ASPARAGUS

This decadent, flavorful low-carb meal will keep you full for hours. The acidity of the roasted red pepper sauce is the perfect counterbalance to the rich steak and pleasing bitterness of the asparagus.

YIELD: 4 servings   PREP TIME: 10 minutes   COOK TIME: 15 to 18 minutes

1 bunch asparagus, about 1 pound

2 tablespoons olive oil, divided, plus more as needed

4 bone-in rib eye steaks, about 8 to 10 ounces each

1 cup roasted piquillo peppers

1 teaspoon smoked paprika

1 clove garlic

1 tablespoon red wine vinegar

sea salt

freshly ground pepper

1. Preheat the oven to 400°F. Line a sheet pan with parchment paper.

2. Add the asparagus to one side of the sheet pan and toss with 1 tablespoon of the olive oil. Season with salt and pepper.

3. Coat the steaks with the remaining tablespoon of olive oil and season generously with salt and pepper. Set them on the other side of the sheet pan.

4. Roast for 10 minutes. Flip the steaks and continue roasting for another 5 to 8 minutes until the steaks are cooked to an internal temperature of 140°F for medium-rare. They will continue cooking after being removed from the pan. Allow the steak to rest for 10 minutes before serving.

5. While the steak and asparagus are roasting, prepare the red pepper sauce by combining the piquillo peppers, smoked paprika, garlic, and red wine vinegar in a blender. Puree until smooth, adding olive oil as needed to round out the sauce. Season with salt and pepper. Serve the sauce over the asparagus with the steaks.

GLUTEN FREE • DAIRY FREE

Nutrition Facts	
(amount per serving)	
Calories	949
Fat	70 g
Protein	72 g
Carbohydrate	8 g
Fiber	3.6 g

BRAISED SHORT RIBS

Beef short ribs have a succulent, fall-off-the-bone texture when slowly roasted with vegetables and wine. The vegetables are used primarily to flavor the sauce, so they do not contribute as many carbs to the recipe as it may appear. For an extra special meal, reduce the pan juices in a small saucepan for a few minutes and whisk in cold butter for a velvety wine sauce.

YIELD: 4 servings   PREP TIME: 10 minutes   COOK TIME: 2 hours

2 pounds beef short ribs, about four 8-ounce short ribs

2 stalks celery, cut into 2-inch pieces

2 carrots, unpeeled, cut into 2-inch pieces

1 red onion, sliced in thick rings

2 thyme sprigs

1 rosemary sprig

1 tablespoon olive oil

½ cup red wine

3 tablespoons cold butter

sea salt

freshly ground pepper

1. Preheat the oven to 375°F.

2. Season the short ribs liberally with salt and pepper. Place them bone-side down on the sheet pan.

3. Scatter the celery, carrot, onion, thyme, and rosemary on the sheet pan and drizzle with the olive oil. Pour in the red wine. Cover the pan tightly with foil and bake for 1½ hours.

4. Remove the pan from the oven and remove the foil. Bake uncovered for another 30 minutes.

5. Transfer the short ribs to a serving platter and cover with foil while you make the sauce.

6. Discard the vegetables and herbs and carefully transfer the pan juices to small saucepan. Bring to a simmer over medium heat until it has reduced in volume to about ½ cup.

7. Remove the pan from the heat and whisk in the butter 1 tablespoon at a time. The sauce will become thick and glossy.

GLUTEN FREE

Nutrition Facts	
(amount per serving)	
Calories	613
Fat	50 g
Protein	31 g
Carbohydrate	4 g
Fiber	1 g

PEPPERCORN-CRUSTED BEEF SHORT RIBS

This impressive dish yields exceptional flavor and a dramatic presentation, making its labor-intensive preparation worth the effort. It looks like it contains a lot of peppercorns, but the gentle simmer in olive oil mellows the flavor and gives it a pleasing amount of spice.

YIELD: 4 servings   PREP TIME: 15 minutes, plus minimum 1 hour inactive time   COOK TIME: 2 hours

1 cup plus 2 tablespoons rainbow peppercorns, divided

1 tablespoon fennel seed

1 tablespoon coriander seed

1 clove garlic, smashed

½ cup sea salt

1 cup boiling water

4 cups ice water

2 pounds beef short ribs

¼ cup olive oil

1 tablespoon red wine vinegar

2 cups baby spinach leaves

1 small bunch radishes, thinly sliced

½ cup pitted Kalamata olives

1 lemon, thinly sliced

1. Toast 2 tablespoons of the peppercorns, fennel, and coriander in a dry skillet until fragrant, about 2 minutes. Transfer them to a large glass dish.

2. Add the garlic clove, sea salt, and 1 cup of boiling water to the dish. Stir until the salt is dissolved. Add another 4 cups of ice water to cool the mixture.

3. Place the short ribs in the brine, meat side down, then cover and brine for at least 1 hour or cover and brine up to 24 hours in the refrigerator.

4. To cook the meat, toast the remaining 1 cup of peppercorns in a dry skillet until fragrant, about 2 minutes. Add the olive oil and simmer over low heat for 30 minutes.

5. Drain excess oil from the peppercorns, reserving it for later. Transfer the peppercorns to a spice grinder and pulverize until it resembles coarse sand.

6. Preheat the oven to 375°F. Line a sheet pan with parchment paper.

7. Remove the meat from the brine and pat dry with paper towels. Coat it with the crushed peppercorns.

8. Place the short ribs on the sheet pan, bone-side down. Cover the pan tightly with foil. Roast for 1½ hours. Remove the foil and roast for another 30 minutes. Allow to rest on the tray for 15 minutes before slicing. Cut the meat away from the bone and into two pieces.

9. Whisk 1 tablespoon of the reserved peppery olive oil with the red wine vinegar in a small bowl.

10. Add the baby spinach, sliced radishes, and olives to the bowl and toss gently to mix. Divide the salad among serving plates and garnish with the lemon slices. Set the short ribs on top of the salad.

GLUTEN FREE · DAIRY FREE

Nutrition Facts	
(amount per serving)	
Calories	704
Fat	66 g
Protein	30 g
Carbohydrate	5 g
Fiber	2.2 g

SOY GINGER SHORT RIBS WITH RED CABBAGE

These Korean-style short ribs for two are perfect to prepare the night before and pop into the oven after a long day of work. The sweet and spicy sriracha, smoky sesame oil, and pungent fish sauce marry beautifully for an addictive sauce. For the ribs, request that your butcher cut them in "flanken-style," which is a method of cutting across the ribs instead of between them (which would be English style).

YIELD: 2 servings   PREP TIME: 15 minutes, plus minimum 1 hour inactive time   COOK TIME: 12 minutes

2 tablespoons soy sauce

2 tablespoons fish sauce

2 tablespoons rice wine vinegar, divided

2 teaspoons sriracha

1 teaspoon sesame oil

2 cloves garlic, minced

1 teaspoon minced fresh ginger

1½ pounds flanken-cut beef short ribs, cut ½-inch thick

2 cups shredded red cabbage

2 scallions, sliced paper thin on a bias

1. Combine the soy sauce, fish sauce, 1 tablespoon of the rice wine vinegar, sriracha, sesame oil, garlic, and ginger in a large glass baking dish or bowl. Add the short ribs meat-side down and marinate in the refrigerator for at least 1 hour or cover and marinate up to 12 hours.

2. Line a sheet pan with foil and top with an oven-safe baking rack. Remove the short ribs from the marinade, shaking off any excess. Pat the ribs dry with a paper towel or, if you have time, allow them to air-dry for 30 minutes. Place the short ribs meat-side up on the rack.

3. Preheat the broiler and place the oven rack on the top level, about 5 inches from the heating element.

4. Broil the short ribs for 5 minutes, then flip over and broil for another 5 minutes. Remove the rack with the ribs to a heat-safe countertop and pour the cabbage onto the pan, tossing to coat in any pan juices.

5. Broil for 1 to 2 minutes or until barely wilted. Season with the remaining rice wine vinegar and garnish with the scallions.

DAIRY FREE

Nutrition Facts	
(amount per serving)	
Calories	795
Fat	71 g
Protein	23 g
Carbohydrate	10 g
Fiber	2.8 g

COWBOY MEATBALLS

These meatballs were one of the most popular recipes from another cookbook I wrote, Sheet Pan Paleo. This version is lower in carbs but still rich in flavor thanks to smoked paprika, minced bacon, and my low-carb Barbecue Sauce (page 212). Bacon in meatballs—who knew?

YIELD: 4 servings   PREP TIME: 10 minutes   COOK TIME: 20 minutes

1 pound ground beef

1 teaspoon sea salt

2 tablespoons flax meal

½ cup minced onion

2 cloves garlic, minced

2 teaspoons smoked paprika

2 slices uncooked bacon, finely chopped

1 egg, whisked

½ cup Barbecue Sauce

1. Preheat the oven to 375°F. Line a sheet pan with parchment paper.

2. Mix the beef, salt, flax meal, onion, garlic, smoked paprika, bacon, and egg in a large bowl and form into 12 to 16 meatballs.

3. Place the meatballs on the sheet pan and bake for 15 minutes.

4. Pour the Barbecue Sauce over the meatballs and return to the oven for another 5 minutes.

GLUTEN FREE · DAIRY FREE · LOW CALORIE

Nutrition Facts	
(amount per serving)	
Calories	435
Fat	34 g
Protein	23 g
Carbohydrate	8 g
Fiber	2 g

BISON BURGERS WITH BACON MAYO

I love the more complex flavor of ground bison, especially when it's married with this smoky Bacon Mayo. If you can't find ground bison, substitute grass-fed beef.

YIELD: 4 servings   PREP TIME: 5 minutes   COOK TIME: 15 to 20 minutes

1 pound ground bison

1 teaspoon minced garlic

1 shallot, minced

½ teaspoon sea salt, divided

¼ teaspoon freshly ground pepper

4 thick slices red onion

1 tablespoon olive oil

8 butter lettuce leaves

½ cup Bacon Mayo (page 204)

4 thick slices tomato

1. Preheat the oven to 375°F. Line a sheet pan with parchment paper.

2. Mix together the bison, garlic, shallot, ¼ teaspoon of the salt, and the pepper. Form into 4 patties and place on the sheet pan.

3. Place the onion slices on the sheet pan and coat in the olive oil and remaining salt.

4. Roast for 15 to 20 minutes or until the burgers are cooked through.

5. To serve, use the butter lettuce leaves as buns and top each burger with a generous dollop of Bacon Mayo and then top with the onions, tomatoes, and another lettuce leaf. Serve immediately.

GLUTEN FREE • DAIRY FREE

Nutrition Facts	
(amount per serving)	
Calories	559
Fat	46 g
Protein	31 g
Carbohydrate	4 g
Fiber	0.7 g

PEPPER JACK BACON CHEESEBURGERS

I got a little carried away with this recipe thinking of all of the typically forbidden foods on most diets—bacon, cheese, and mayonnaise. Roasting the onions and tomatoes brings out their natural sweetness while keeping the carbs ultra-low.

YIELD: 4 servings   PREP TIME: 5 minutes   COOK TIME: 15 minutes

1 pound ground beef

½ teaspoon sea salt, divided

¼ teaspoon freshly ground pepper

4 thick slices red onion

4 thick slices tomato

1 tablespoon olive oil

4 slices Pepper Jack cheese

8 butter lettuce leaves

¼ cup mayonnaise

4 slices thick-cut cooked bacon

1. Preheat the oven to 375°F. Line a sheet pan with parchment paper.

2. Season the ground beef with ¼ teaspoon of the salt and the pepper. Form into 4 patties and place on the sheet pan.

3. Place the onion and tomato slices on the sheet pan and coat in the olive oil and remaining salt.

4. Roast for 10 minutes, then flip the burgers and top each one with 1 slice of cheese. Cook for another 5 minutes or until the burgers are cooked through and the cheese is melted.

5. To serve, use the butter lettuce leaves as buns and smear ½ tablespoon of mayonnaise on each leaf. Place a burger patty in four of the lettuce leaves and top each burger with the bacon, roasted tomatoes and onion, and another lettuce leaf. Serve immediately.

GLUTEN FREE

Nutrition Facts	
(amount per serving)	
Calories	533
Fat	45 g
Protein	26 g
Carbohydrate	4 g
Fiber	0.6 g

RIB EYE STEAK AND PEPPER FAJITAS

The fat from the steak renders during the roasting to flavor the onions and peppers. Serve this filling with low-carb wraps or butter lettuce leaves.

YIELD: 6 servings   PREP TIME: 10 minutes   COOK TIME: 20 minutes

1 tablespoon smoked paprika

1 teaspoon ground coriander

1 tablespoon ground cumin

1¼ teaspoons sea salt, divided

2 boneless rib eye steaks, about 8 ounces each

2 tablespoons olive oil, divided

2 bell peppers, assorted colors, cut into 1-inch slices

1 yellow onion, halved then sliced in half circles

freshly ground pepper

1 head butter lettuce

1 cup shredded sharp cheddar cheese

1 large avocado, cut into thin slices

½ cup roughly chopped fresh cilantro (optional)

½ cup full-fat sour cream

1. Preheat the oven to 400°F. Line a sheet pan with parchment paper.

2. Combine the paprika, coriander, cumin, and 1 teaspoon of the salt in a small bowl. Pat the steaks dry with paper towels and then coat with 1 tablespoon of the olive oil. Press the spice rub into the meat. If you prepare it ahead of time, you can simply set it uncovered in the refrigerator.

3. Spread the peppers and onion on the sheet pan and toss with the remaining olive oil and season with pepper and the remaining sea salt.

4. Set the steaks in the center of the pan, surrounding each one with the onion and pepper mixture. Roast for 20 minutes or until the tenderloin reaches an internal temperature of 145°F. Allow the meat to rest for 10 minutes before slicing thinly.

5. To serve, fill a butter lettuce leaf with a few slices of beef and a spoonful of peppers and onions. Top with a pinch of shredded cheese, avocado, cilantro, and sour cream.

GLUTEN FREE

Nutrition Facts	
(amount per serving)	
Calories	767
Fat	64 g
Protein	43 g
Carbohydrate	10 g
Fiber	4.1 g

ASIAN FLANK STEAK LETTUCE WRAPS

These lettuce wraps are a cinch to prepare in advance. Simply allow them to marinate, then throw together in a few minutes. They're especially great for meal planning.

YIELD: 4 servings   PREP TIME: 10 minutes, plus minimum 1 hour inactive time   COOK TIME: 10 minutes

¼ cup rice wine vinegar

½ cup boiling water

1 tablespoon sea salt

1 teaspoon red chile flakes

1 tablespoon minced ginger

1 tablespoon minced garlic

1 cup ice water

1½ pounds flank steak

1 tablespoon toasted sesame oil

1 head butter lettuce

¼ cup minced red onions

½ cup roughly chopped fresh cilantro

½ cup roughly chopped dry roasted peanuts

sea salt

freshly ground black pepper

1. Combine the vinegar, boiling water, salt, red chile flakes, ginger, and garlic in a large shallow dish. Stir until the salt is dissolved. Add the ice water. Marinate the flank steak for 1 hour or cover and marinate up to 8 hours in the refrigerator.

2. To cook the steak, preheat the broiler.

3. Remove the meat from the marinade and pat dry with paper towels. Place on a sheet pan and rub with the sesame oil. Season with salt and pepper.

4. Place under the broiler for 5 minutes, then turn to the other side and broil for another 5 minutes or until it reaches your desired level of doneness. Allow the meat to rest for 10 minutes before slicing.

5. To serve, fill each lettuce leaf with a few slices of meat. Top with red onions, cilantro, and peanuts.

GLUTEN FREE ▪ DAIRY FREE ▪ LOW CALORIE

Nutrition Facts	
(amount per serving)	
Calories	417
Fat	25 g
Protein	40 g
Carbohydrate	8 g
Fiber	2.5 g

CARNE ASADA LETTUCE WRAPS

Take the Asian Flank Steak Lettuce Wraps (page 172) in a Latin direction with this simple, spicy marinade. Serve with fresh guacamole, or for an even simpler option, use sliced avocado.

YIELD: 4 servings   PREP TIME: 10 minutes, plus minimum 1 hour inactive time   COOK TIME: 10 minutes

juice of 1 lime

2 tablespoons olive oil

2 teaspoons ground cumin

2 teaspoons minced fresh oregano

2 teaspoons ancho chile powder

½ teaspoon sea salt

½ teaspoon freshly ground pepper

1½ pounds flank steak

1 head butter lettuce

1 small red onion, thinly sliced

½ cup fresh cilantro, for serving

1 cup Guacamole (page 206)

1. Combine the lime juice, olive oil, cumin, oregano, ancho chile powder, sea salt, and pepper in a small bowl. Coat the flank steak in the mixture and allow to rest for 5 minutes at room temperature, or cover and place in the refrigerator for up to 8 hours.

2. To cook the meat, preheat the broiler.

3. Remove the meat from the marinade and place on a sheet pan. Place under the broiler for 5 minutes, then turn to the other side and broil for another 5 minutes or until it reaches your desired level of doneness. Allow the meat to rest for 10 minutes before slicing.

4. To serve, fill each lettuce leaf with a few slices of meat. Top with red onions, cilantro, and Guacamole.

GLUTEN FREE ▪ DAIRY FREE ▪ LOW CALORIE

Nutrition Facts	
(amount per serving)	
Calories	446
Fat	24 g
Protein	37 g
Carbohydrate	8 g
Fiber	3.2 g

PRIME RIB ROAST

Save this succulent prime rib roast for special occasions. It can serve a crowd and makes excellent leftovers. See below for three variations on how to use up those leftovers.

YIELD: 10 servings   PREP TIME: 10 minutes, plus 8 hours inactive time
COOK TIME: 1½ to 2 hours

2 tablespoons minced garlic

1 tablespoon minced rosemary

1 teaspoon sea salt

1 teaspoon freshly ground pepper

3 tablespoons olive oil

1 center-cut prime rib roast, 3 to 4 pounds

1. Combine the garlic, rosemary, sea salt, pepper, and olive oil. Coat the rib roast in this mixture and place in the refrigerator uncovered for 8 hours or overnight.

2. Remove the meat from the refrigerator at least 1 hour before placing in the oven.

3. Preheat the oven to 450°F. Place the meat on a sheet pan and roast uncovered for 30 minutes to develop a nice crust on the exterior.

4. Reduce the heat to 325°F. Roast for another 1 to 1½ hours or until the roast reaches an internal temperature of 140°F. Remove to a cutting board and allow to rest for 20 minutes before slicing and serving.

GLUTEN FREE ▪ DAIRY FREE ▪ LOW CALORIE

Nutrition Facts	
(amount per serving)	
Calories	413
Fat	25 g
Protein	43 g
Carbohydrate	0 g
Fiber	0 g

SALSA VERDE PRIME RIB WRAPS

Make the recipe for Prime Rib Roast. Place one serving of prime rib into one low-carb wrap and top with ¼ cup of Salsa Verde (page 207).

GLUTEN FREE · DAIRY FREE

Nutrition Facts	
(amount per serving)	
Calories	608
Fat	44 g
Protein	44 g
Carbohydrate	8 g
Fiber	2.2 g

PRIME RIB STIR-FRY

1. Make the recipe for Prime Rib Roast.

2. Heat 1 tablespoon toasted sesame oil over medium-high heat. Stir fry 1 cup broccoli until crisp-tender, about 5 to 7 minutes.

3. Add 1 teaspoon minced garlic, 1 teaspoon minced ginger, and a pinch of red chile flakes to the pan. Cook for 30 seconds.

4. Add 1 serving of Prime Rib Roast to the pan and cook briefly, until barely heated through.

5. Add 2 tablespoons soy sauce to the pan and 1 teaspoon rice wine vinegar. Cook for 30 seconds and then serve.

GLUTEN FREE · DAIRY FREE

Nutrition Facts	
(amount per serving)	
Calories	556
Fat	40 g
Protein	44 g
Carbohydrate	4 g
Fiber	2.2 g

PRIME RIB CAULI-RICE BOWLS

Make the recipe for Prime Rib Roast. Place 1 serving of prime rib over 1 serving Cauliflower Rice (page 220) and top with 2 tablespoons Guacamole (page 206) and 2 tablespoons roasted tomato salsa.

GLUTEN FREE ▪ DAIRY FREE

Nutrition Facts	
(amount per serving)	
Calories	541
Fat	33 g
Protein	47 g
Carbohydrate	13 g
Fiber	5.6 g

SHEET PAN KETOGENIC

ROSEMARY ORANGE RIB EYE STEAKS

This is the type of dish everyone thinks of when they think "low-carb diet"—nothing but meat and butter. But this dish is so much more! Orange, rosemary, and black pepper infuse the steaks with flavor. If you prefer not to make your own compound butter, most well-stocked grocery stores have flavorful options in the dairy case.

YIELD: 4 servings   PREP TIME: 5 minutes   COOK TIME: 15 to 17 minutes

4 bone-in rib eye steaks, about 6 ounces each

1 tablespoon canola oil

sea salt

freshly ground pepper

1 stick (½ cup) Rosemary Orange Compound Butter (page 201)

1. Preheat the oven to 450°F. Place the sheet pan in the oven while it preheats.

2. Pat the steaks dry with paper towels and then rub the meat with canola oil and season with salt and pepper.

3. Place the steaks on the hot sheet pan and roast for 10 minutes. Remove the pan from the oven and flip the steaks. Top the steaks with a thick slice of the compound butter (about 2 tablespoons per steak). Return the pan to the oven and cook for another 5 to 7 minutes for medium-rare.

GLUTEN FREE

Nutrition Facts	
(amount per serving)	
Calories	998
Fat	90 g
Protein	54 g
Carbohydrate	0 g
Fiber	0 g

BEEF AND VEGETABLE KEBABS

Take these basic beef and vegetable kebabs in a variety of directions. Feeling Middle Eastern cuisine? Serve with olives, tahini, and cucumbers. Feeling like Mexican food? Opt for a generous dollop of guacamole and sour cream. They also make great filling for low-carb wraps.

YIELD: 4 servings   PREP TIME: 10 minutes   COOK TIME: 15 to 20 minutes

24 ounces boneless rib eye steak, cut into 1-inch pieces

1 red bell pepper, cored and cut into 1-inch pieces

1 green bell pepper, cored and cut into 1-inch pieces

1 small red onion, cut into 1-inch pieces

2 tablespoons canola oil

sea salt

freshly ground pepper

1. Preheat the oven to 400°F.

2. Thread the steak, bell peppers, and onion onto skewers. Set them onto the sheet pan. Brush with canola oil and season with salt and pepper.

3. Bake for 15 to 20 minutes or until the steak is cooked through and the vegetables are soft.

GLUTEN FREE · DAIRY FREE · LOW CALORIE

Nutrition Facts	
(amount per serving)	
Calories	348
Fat	19 g
Protein	37 g
Carbohydrate	5 g
Fiber	1.3 g

SHEET PAN KETOGENIC

BEEF AND VEGETABLE KEBABS WITH OLIVES, TAHINI, AND CUCUMBER

Make the Beef and Vegetable Kebabs and serve with 1 cup assorted olives and 1 cucumber cut into spears. Serve with ¼ cup tahini for dipping.

GLUTEN FREE • DAIRY FREE • LOW CALORIE

Nutrition Facts	
(amount per serving)	
Calories	466
Fat	29 g
Protein	40 g
Carbohydrate	10 g
Fiber	3.3 g

CHIPOTLE BEEF AND VEGETABLE KEBABS WITH GUACAMOLE

Make the Beef and Vegetable Kebabs and season with 1 tablespoon ground chipotle powder. Serve with 1 cup Guacamole (page 206).

GLUTEN FREE • DAIRY FREE • LOW CALORIE

Nutrition Facts	
(amount per serving)	
Calories	448
Fat	28 g
Protein	38 g
Carbohydrate	11 g
Fiber	4.3 g

LAMB MEATBALL WRAPS WITH TZATZIKI

Full-flavored ground lamb spiked with oregano, thyme, and fresh garlic is balanced with cool, creamy tzatziki sauce in these tasty wraps.

YIELD: 4 servings   PREP TIME: 10 minutes   COOK TIME: 15 minutes

1 pound ground lamb

1 teaspoon sea salt

2 tablespoons flax meal

½ cup minced onion

2 cloves garlic, minced

1 tablespoon dried oregano

1 teaspoon dried thyme

1 egg, whisked

4 low-carb wraps, such as NUCO

1 cup Tzatziki (page 205)

1 plum tomato, diced

1. Preheat the oven to 375°F. Line a sheet pan with parchment paper.

2. Mix the lamb, salt, flax meal, onion, garlic, oregano, thyme, and egg in a large bowl and form into 12 to 16 meatballs.

3. Place the meatballs on the sheet pan and bake for 15 minutes until browned and cooked all the way through.

4. Serve 3 to 4 meatballs in each wrap and top with Tzatziki and a sprinkle of diced tomatoes.

GLUTEN FREE

Nutrition Facts	
(amount per serving)	
Calories	518
Fat	34 g
Protein	23 g
Carbohydrate	7 g
Fiber	1.5 g

CHAPTER NINE

Desserts

Even on a low-carb diet, it's nice to finish a meal with a little something sweet. These decadent desserts are lightly sweetened with stevia. Unlike other keto desserts, these are not designed to be carb free. It is dessert after all! But, you will be pleasantly surprised at how yummy these treats are while keeping the carbs to a minimum.

CHOCOLATE CHIP COOKIES

This was one of the first recipes I learned to cook by myself. By the time I graduated high school, I had the recipe down to a science. Unfortunately, it had equal parts sugar and flour, not to mention heaps of chocolate chips, making these cookies little carb bombs. My new version uses almond flour and liquid stevia for a much lighter, but equally delicious, version. They taste so good, they even wowed my son's third grade class when I brought in a batch during recipe testing! Look for extra-dark chocolate chips or use a sugar-free version.

YIELD: 12 servings   PREP TIME: 5 minutes   COOK TIME: 10 minutes

2 cups almond flour	2 tablespoons almond milk
1 teaspoon baking powder	1 tablespoon vanilla extract
½ teaspoon sea salt	½ teaspoon liquid stevia
3 tablespoons coconut oil	½ cup dark chocolate chips, at least 60% cacao

1. Preheat the oven to 350°F. Line a sheet pan with parchment paper.

2. Combine the almond flour, baking powder, and sea salt in a large bowl.

3. Stir in the coconut oil.

4. Combine the milk, vanilla extract, and stevia in a separate container and then pour into the bowl with the flour and coconut oil mixture. Stir to mix thoroughly.

5. Fold in the chocolate chips.

6. Form the dough into 12 balls and place on the sheet pan. Flatten them gently with your hand; they will not spread during baking.

7. Bake for 10 minutes and then transfer to a cooling rack. Store in a covered container in the refrigerator for up to 3 days or in the freezer for up to 1 month.

GLUTEN FREE ▪ VEGETARIAN ▪ DAIRY FREE ▪ LOW CALORIE

SHEET PAN KETOGENIC

Nutrition Facts	
(amount per serving)	
Calories	166
Fat	15 g
Protein	4 g
Carbohydrate	7 g
Fiber	2.3 g

TIP: This cookie is crafted to be dairy free. But, if you prefer to use butter and milk, use them in place of the coconut oil and almond milk.

SALTY SWEET PEANUT BUTTER COOKIES

If you scan the ingredients list, you'll see that I included 1 teaspoon of real sugar. The sacrilege! Hear me out. The peanut butter cookies I grew up with had a fine, crunchy layer of sugar on the top. In this recipe, a tiny amount of sugar, along with salt, functions as a finishing element and it adds a fraction of a gram of carbohydrate to each cookie.

YIELD: 24 servings   PREP TIME: 10 minutes   COOK TIME: 10 minutes

1 cup creamy natural peanut butter

1 stick (½ cup) butter, softened

2 eggs

1½ teaspoons liquid stevia

1 teaspoon vanilla extract

2 cups almond flour

¼ teaspoon baking soda

1¼ teaspoons sea salt, divided

1 teaspoon granulated sugar (optional)

1. Preheat the oven to 350°F. Line a baking sheet with parchment paper.

2. Using an electric mixer, cream the peanut butter and butter until thoroughly integrated.

3. Add the eggs, stevia, and vanilla and beat for 30 seconds, scraping down the sides of the bowl once.

4. Sift in the almond flour, baking powder, and ¼ teaspoon of salt into the bowl. Stir until just combined.

5. Form the dough into 12 balls and place them onto the sheet pan.

6. Combine the remaining teaspoon of salt and granulated sugar in a small dish. Dip the tines of a fork into the sugar and salt mixture and then use the fork to flatten each cookie, making two perpendicular press marks.

7. Bake for 10 minutes and then transfer to a cooling rack. Store in a covered container in the refrigerator for up to 3 days or in the freezer for up to 1 month.

GLUTEN FREE ▪ VEGETARIAN ▪ LOW CALORIE

Nutrition Facts	
(amount per serving)	
Calories	158
Fat	14 g
Protein	5 g
Carbohydrate	4 g
Fiber	1.6 g

ALL-BUTTER SHORTBREAD

Butter is so delicious you might want to eat it by itself, but here's a much tastier way to get your fix. These shortbreads are crumbly and delicious and go well with a cup of bulletproof coffee.

YIELD: 32 (2¼ x 2½-inch) servings   PREP TIME: 5 minutes
COOK TIME: 10 to 12 minutes

4 cups almond flour	¼ cup half-and-half
1 teaspoon baking powder	1 tablespoon vanilla extract
1 teaspoon sea salt	1½ teaspoons liquid stevia
1 stick (½ cup) butter, softened	

1. Preheat the oven to 350°F. Line a sheet pan with parchment paper.

2. Combine the almond flour, baking powder, and sea salt in a large bowl.

3. Stir in the butter.

4. Combine the half-and-half, vanilla extract, and stevia in a small bowl and then pour into the bowl with the flour and butter mixture. Stir to mix thoroughly.

5. Spread the dough out onto the sheet pan. Form a small square or spread it all the way to the edges for thin shortbread.

6. Bake for 10 to 12 minutes and then transfer the pan to a cooling rack. Cut into 32 pieces, about 2¼ x 2½ inches each. Store in a covered container in the refrigerator for up to 3 days or in the freezer for up to 1 month.

GLUTEN FREE ▪ VEGETARIAN ▪ LOW CALORIE

Nutrition Facts	
(amount per serving)	
Calories	109
Fat	10 g
Protein	3 g
Carbohydrate	3 g
Fiber	1.5 g

APPLE STREUSEL BARS

Cinnamon and apple are a classic combination, but did you know that eating cinnamon may improve blood sugar levels over time by lowering insulin resistance? This is welcome news if you're looking to a low-carb diet to address symptoms of pre-diabetes. But any excuse to eat more cinnamon is good in my book!

YIELD: 48 (1 ½ x 2½-inch) servings   PREP TIME: 10 minutes
COOK TIME: 20 to 25 minutes

3 cups almond flour

1 cup coconut flour

1 teaspoon sea salt

2 teaspoons liquid stevia

1 tablespoon vanilla extract

1 cup butter or coconut oil, softened

2 eggs

1 cup no-sugar-added apple butter

1 tablespoon ground cinnamon

2 cups roughly chopped, toasted pecans

1. Preheat the oven to 350°F. Line a sheet pan with parchment paper.

2. Combine the almond flour, coconut flour, sea salt, stevia, and vanilla in a large bowl.

3. Stir in the butter or oil and egg until thoroughly combined.

4. Reserve 1½ cups of this crust mixture for the topping. Transfer the remaining crust to the sheet pan and press it into the pan with your hands, spreading to the edges.

5. Spread the apple butter over the top of the crust.

6. Combine the reserved crust mixture with the ground cinnamon and pecans and mix with your hands. Crumble the mixture over the pan.

7. Bake for 20 to 25 minutes or until the topping begins to brown. Allow to cool completely before slicing. Cut into 48 bars, about 1½ x 2½ inches each.

GLUTEN FREE • VEGETARIAN • LOW CALORIE

Nutrition Facts
(amount per serving)

Calories	128
Fat	11.5 g
Protein	3 g
Carbohydrate	5 g
Fiber	3 g

RASPBERRY CREAM CHEESE BARS

I enjoyed a breakfast coffee cake with this flavor combination and was undone, not only with the flavors but with how cloying it was. I instantly felt the sugar rush and regretted the indulgence. My new version has all the delicious raspberry and almond flavors of the original, without any refined sugar or flour.

YIELD: 48 (1½ x 2½-inch) servings   PREP TIME: 10 minutes
COOK TIME: 20 to 25 minutes

3 cups almond flour

1 cup coconut flour

1 teaspoon sea salt

2 teaspoons liquid stevia

1 tablespoon vanilla extract

¼ teaspoon almond extract

2 sticks (1 cup) butter, softened

2 eggs

1 cup no-sugar added raspberry jam

16 ounces cold cream cheese

2 cups toasted thinly sliced almonds

1. Preheat the oven to 350°F. Line a sheet pan with parchment paper.

2. Combine the almond flour, coconut flour, sea salt, stevia, vanilla, and almond extract in a large bowl. Mix in the butter and eggs and stir until thoroughly combined.

3. Reserve 1 cup of this crust mixture for the topping. Transfer the remaining crust to the sheet pan and press it into the pan with your hands, spreading to the edges.

4. Spread the raspberry jam over the top of the crust.

5. Using a sharp knife, thinly slice the cream cheese, as if slicing regular cheese for a sandwich. Spread these slices evenly over the raspberry layer.

6. Crumble the reserved crust over the cheese layer and then sprinkle with the almonds.

7. Bake for 20 to 25 minutes or until the topping begins to brown. Allow to cool completely before slicing. Cut into 48 bars, about 1½ x 2½ inches each.

GLUTEN FREE ▪ VEGETARIAN ▪ LOW CALORIE

Nutrition Facts	
(amount per serving)	
Calories	150
Fat	13.5 g
Protein	4 g
Carbohydrate	6 g
Fiber	2.7 g

SLAB PUMPKIN PIE

Top this rich autumn-spiced pumpkin pie with whipped heavy cream for an especially decadent dessert, or even breakfast. (I may have done this once or twice!) Make sure to purchase 100 percent pure pumpkin puree that has not been sweetened with added sugar.

YIELD: 48 (1½ x 2½-inch) servings   PREP TIME: 15 minutes
COOK TIME: 45 to 50 minutes

For the crust:

4 cups almond flour

¼ cup coconut flour

1 teaspoon sea salt

1 stick (½ cup) butter, cold, cut into small cubes

2 eggs

2 tablespoons heavy cream

¼ teaspoon liquid stevia

ice water, as needed

For the filling:

2 cups heavy cream

4 cups pumpkin puree

4 eggs

2 teaspoons liquid stevia, plus more to taste

2 tablespoons pumpkin pie spice

¾ teaspoon sea salt

1. Preheat the oven to 350°F. Measure two sheets of parchment paper that are slightly larger than your sheet pan to allow the paper to go up on all sides.

2. To make the crust, combine the almond flour, coconut flour, and sea salt. Cut the butter in using a pastry cutter until the mixture resembles breadcrumbs. (Or, use your food processor to do this.)

3. Add the eggs, heavy cream, and stevia to the crust and stir until barely combined. There should still be chunks of butter remaining. Add a teaspoon or two of ice water, if needed, until the mixture begins to come together. Wrap the dough in plastic and refrigerate while you make the filling.

4. To make the filling, whisk together the heavy cream, pumpkin puree, eggs, stevia, pumpkin pie spice, and sea salt.

5. Remove the chilled crust, place the dough on one sheet of parchment paper, and top with the second sheet. Roll the crust out until it nearly reaches the edges of the paper. Peel away the top sheet of parchment and carefully slide the bottom sheet onto the pan. Gently press the crust into the corners of the pan.

6. Pour the filling mixture into the sheet pan and carefully transfer it to the oven. Bake for 45 to 50 minutes or until the pie is almost completely set. It will still be slightly jiggly in the very center. Allow to cool at room temperature and then chill in the refrigerator for at least 1 hour until ready to serve. Cut into 48 bars, about 1½ x 2½ inches each.

GLUTEN FREE ▪ VEGETARIAN ▪ LOW CALORIE

Nutrition Facts	
(amount per serving)	
Calories	126
Fat	11.5 g
Protein	3.5 g
Carbohydrate	4.5 g
Fiber	2.2 g

SLAB CHEESECAKE FOUR WAYS

Is there anything more scrumptious than cheesecake? Yes—knowing you're only getting 4 grams or less of carbs per serving! I developed this crust that uses freshly ground roasted hazelnuts and a generous amount of sea salt held together with butter. To me, it tastes just like a graham cracker crust. If you prefer a traditional piecrust, use the crust in Slab Pumpkin Pie (page 194).

YIELD: 48 (1½ x 2½-inch) servings   PREP TIME: 15 minutes
COOK TIME: 50 to 60 minutes

For the crust:

4 cups finely ground toasted hazelnuts

1½ teaspoons sea salt

4 tablespoons butter, melted

¼ teaspoon liquid stevia

For the cheesecake:

32 ounces full-fat cream cheese (4 packages), softened

1 cup sour cream

4 eggs

1 tablespoon vanilla extract

2 teaspoons liquid stevia

1. Preheat the oven to 400°F. Measure one sheet of parchment paper that is slightly larger than your sheet pan to allow the paper to go up on all sides. Press it into the pan.

2. To make the crust, combine the ground hazelnuts and sea salt in a large bowl. Drizzle in the butter and stevia, and mix.

3. Press the hazelnut crust into the pan using a fork or your hands.

4. Bake for 10 minutes. Remove the pan from the oven and turn the heat down to 300°F.

5. To make the filling, beat the cream cheese, sour cream, eggs, vanilla extract, and stevia in a large bowl.

6. Pour the filling mixture into the sheet pan and carefully transfer it to the oven. Bake for 40 to 50 minutes or until the cheesecake is set and beginning to brown around the edges. Allow to cool at room temperature and then chill in the refrigerator for at least 2 hours until ready to serve. Cut into 48 bars, about 1½ x 2½ inches each.

GLUTEN FREE ▪ VEGETARIAN ▪ LOW CALORIE

Nutrition Facts	
(amount per serving)	
Calories	143
Fat	14 g
Protein	3.5 g
Carbohydrate	2.5 g
Fiber	.8 g

CHERRY SWIRL CHEESECAKE

Before baking, drop 1 cup of sugar-free cherry preserves by the tablespoon onto the cheesecake. Swirl with a knife. Bake as usual.

GLUTEN FREE ▪ VEGETARIAN ▪ LOW CALORIE

Nutrition Facts	
(amount per serving)	
Calories	146
Fat	14 g
Protein	3.5 g
Carbohydrate	4 g
Fiber	.8 g

PEANUT BUTTER FUDGE CHEESECAKE

Mix 1 cup creamy natural peanut butter and ½ cup melted chocolate chips into the filling. Bake as usual.

GLUTEN FREE ▪ VEGETARIAN ▪ LOW CALORIE

Nutrition Facts	
(amount per serving)	
Calories	181
Fat	17 g
Protein	5 g
Carbohydrate	4 g
Fiber	1.2 g

CHOCOLATE ESPRESSO SWIRL CHEESECAKE

Add 2 tablespoons instant espresso powder to the filling. Pour into the prepared crust. Melt ½ cup extra-dark chocolate chips and drizzle over the cheesecake. Swirl with a knife. Bake as usual.

GLUTEN FREE ▪ VEGETARIAN ▪ LOW CALORIE

Nutrition Facts	
(amount per serving)	
Calories	149
Fat	14.5 g
Protein	3.5 g
Carbohydrate	3.1 g
Fiber	1 g

CHAPTER TEN

Sauces, Dips, and Other Extras

Sometimes you want a little something extra to go with your meal. Here are recipes for sauces, dips, and salads to accompany your sheet pan meals. They're a great way to sneak a little more fat into a recipe, especially if you want to alter the ratio of protein to fat. They're also a fun way to add new colors and textures—think bright and crunchy—without upping your carbs too much.

GARLIC HERB COMPOUND BUTTER

This may be your new favorite low-carb food. Okay, not by itself, but this compound butter is loaded with all of the delectable flavor of butter infused with herbs, lemon, and garlic. Branch out and try your new flavor combinations with the variations that follow. They are perfect added to steak, seafood, or poultry.

YIELD: 8 (1-tablespoon) servings   PREP TIME: 10 minutes
COOK TIME: none

1 stick (½ cup) butter, softened

1 tablespoon minced fresh parsley

1 tablespoon minced fresh mint

1 teaspoon minced garlic

1 teaspoon lemon zest

Mash the butter with the desired spices until thoroughly integrated. Place it on a square of plastic wrap or parchment paper and shape it into a log. Roll and seal tightly. Store in the refrigerator for up to 1 week or in the freezer for up to 1 month.

GLUTEN FREE · VEGETARIAN · LOW CALORIE

Nutrition Facts	
(amount per serving)	
Calories	102
Fat	12 g
Protein	0 g
Carbohydrate	0 g
Fiber	0 g

SMOKY GARLIC COMPOUND BUTTER

Begin with 1 stick softened butter and add 1 tablespoon minced cilantro, 1 teaspoon minced garlic, 1 teaspoon ground chipotle, and 1 teaspoon smoked paprika.

GLUTEN FREE ▪ VEGETARIAN ▪ LOW CALORIE

Nutrition Facts	
(amount per serving)	
Calories	102
Fat	12 g
Protein	0 g
Carbohydrate	0 g
Fiber	0 g

ROSEMARY ORANGE COMPOUND BUTTER

Begin with 1 stick softened butter and add 1 tablespoon minced fresh rosemary, 1 teaspoon finely grated orange zest, and ¼ teaspoon freshly ground black pepper.

GLUTEN FREE ▪ VEGETARIAN ▪ LOW CALORIE

Nutrition Facts	
(amount per serving)	
Calories	102
Fat	12 g
Protein	0 g
Carbohydrate	0 g
Fiber	0 g

TARRAGON COMPOUND BUTTER

Begin with 1 stick softened butter and add 2 tablespoons minced tarragon, 2 tablespoons grated Parmesan cheese, and 1 tablespoon minced shallot.

GLUTEN FREE · VEGETARIAN · LOW CALORIE

Nutrition Facts	
(amount per serving)	
Calories	102
Fat	12 g
Protein	0 g
Carbohydrate	0 g
Fiber	0 g

CAPER DILL COMPOUND BUTTER

Begin with 1 stick softened butter and add 1 tablespoon minced dill, 1 tablespoon minced scallions, and 1 teaspoon minced capers.

GLUTEN FREE · VEGETARIAN · LOW CALORIE

Nutrition Facts	
(amount per serving)	
Calories	102
Fat	12 g
Protein	0 g
Carbohydrate	0 g
Fiber	0 g

HOLLANDAISE SAUCE

This decadent, buttery sauce is the low-carb dieter's best friend. Use it as a dipping sauce for Avocado Bacon Fries (page 43) or pour it over simple roasted asparagus.

YIELD: 4 (2-tablespoon) servings   PREP TIME: 5 minutes
COOK TIME: 2 minutes

8 tablespoons cold butter, divided

2 egg yolks

1½ teaspoons lemon juice

1½ teaspoons cold water

pinch sea salt

1. Melt 7 tablespoons of the butter in a microwave-safe dish.

2. In a small skillet, whisk the egg yolks thoroughly and then add the lemon juice, water, and salt.

3. Turn the heat to low and cook the egg yolk mixture for about 2 minutes until thick and warm.

4. Whisk in 1 tablespoon of the cold butter to cool the mixture.

5. Slowly drizzle in the melted butter, whisking constantly until it is all incorporated and the sauce is thick and smooth.

6. Serve immediately, as the sauce does not keep or reheat well.

GLUTEN FREE ▪ VEGETARIAN ▪ LOW CALORIE

Nutrition Facts	
(amount per serving)	
Calories	232
Fat	25 g
Protein	2 g
Carbohydrate	1 g
Fiber	0 g

BACON MAYO

I followed a Paleo-style diet for a few years and enjoyed more than my fair share of bacon. I didn't always need the rendered fat from cooked bacon and had to get creative for using it up. Enter: bacon mayo. This thick, creamy mayonnaise is, as they say, awesome sauce. Use it on Bison Burgers (page 167) or as a base for other sauces. Thanks to the saturated fat in the bacon, this sauce becomes solid when stored in the refrigerator, so plan to make it just before you want to use it.

YIELD: 8 (1-tablespoon) servings   PREP TIME: 5 minutes
COOK TIME: none

1 egg yolk

½ teaspoon lemon juice

pinch sea salt

½ cup rendered bacon fat, melted but not hot

1. Whisk the egg yolk, lemon juice, and sea salt in a small bowl for about 30 seconds.

2. Slowly drizzle in the bacon fat a drop or two at a time, whisking constantly. The mixture will thicken as you add the fat. Keep whisking until it is all incorporated.

GLUTEN FREE ▪ DAIRY FREE ▪ LOW CALORIE

Nutrition Facts	
(amount per serving)	
Calories	122
Fat	13 g
Protein	0 g
Carbohydrate	0 g
Fiber	0 g

TZATZIKI

Serve this tangy yogurt-based sauce with Lamb Meatball Wraps (page 182).

YIELD: 6 (¼-cup) servings   PREP TIME: 5 minutes   COOK TIME: none

1 cup full-fat yogurt

½ cup full-fat mayonnaise

½ cup finely diced, peeled cucumber

1 teaspoon minced fresh garlic

1 tablespoon minced fresh dill

sea salt

freshly ground pepper

Whisk the yogurt, mayonnaise, cucumber, garlic, and dill in a small bowl. Season with salt and pepper.

GLUTEN FREE · VEGETARIAN · LOW CALORIE

Nutrition Facts	
(amount per serving)	
Calories	147
Fat	15 g
Protein	2 g
Carbohydrate	2 g
Fiber	0.1 g

GUACAMOLE

This zesty guacamole is loaded with healthy monounsaturated fats. It is delicious with scrambled eggs, Shrimp Fajita Bowls (page 78) and Rib Eye Steak and Pepper Fajitas (page 170).

YIELD: 8 (2-tablespoon) servings   PREP TIME: 5 minutes
COOK TIME: none

1 cup mashed avocado, from about 4 small avocados

1 shallot, minced

1 jalapeno pepper, minced

1 tablespoon lime juice

sea salt

freshly ground pepper

Combine all of the ingredients in a medium bowl or mortar and pestle. Cover and refrigerate until ready to serve.

GLUTEN FREE ▪ VEGETARIAN ▪ DAIRY FREE ▪ LOW CALORIE

Nutrition Facts	
(amount per serving)	
Calories	50
Fat	4.4 g
Protein	6 g
Carbohydrate	3 g
Fiber	2 g

SALSA VERDE

This punchy green salsa is amazing on Salsa Verde Shrimp (page 77) or served as a condiment on pretty much anything, especially Carne Asada Lettuce Wraps (page 174).

YIELD: 4 (¼-cup) servings   PREP TIME: 5 minutes   COOK TIME: none

1 cup loosely packed fresh cilantro

1 jalapeno pepper, cored and roughly chopped

2 cloves garlic, roughly chopped

juice of 1 lime

¼ cup extra-virgin olive oil

¼ teaspoon sea salt

Place all ingredients in a blender and puree until mostly smooth. Serve immediately or store in a covered container for up to 3 days in the refrigerator.

GLUTEN FREE • VEGETARIAN • DAIRY FREE • LOW CALORIE

Nutrition Facts	
(amount per serving)	
Calories	125
Fat	14 g
Protein	0 g
Carbohydrate	2 g
Fiber	0.2 g

RANCH DIP

This easy ranch dip recipe is perfect with Avocado Bacon Fries (page 43) or Fiery Chicken Wings (page 44), or thin it with a little more buttermilk to make a ranch dressing for green salads.

YIELD: 12 (2-tablespoon) servings   PREP TIME: 5 minutes
COOK TIME: none

2 tablespoons minced fresh parsley

1 teaspoon minced fresh dill

2 cloves garlic, minced

1 shallot, minced

1 cup full-fat mayonnaise

½ cup buttermilk

sea salt

freshly ground pepper

Combine the parsley, dill, garlic, shallot, mayonnaise, and buttermilk in a small bowl. Season with salt and pepper. Store in a covered container in the refrigerator for up to 3 days.

GLUTEN FREE ▪ VEGETARIAN ▪ LOW CALORIE

Nutrition Facts	
(amount per serving)	
Calories	127
Fat	13 g
Protein	1 g
Carbohydrate	1 g
Fiber	0 g

PESTO

Most commercially prepared pesto contains Parmesan cheese, and while it does add a deliciously nutty flavor, if you find dairy difficult to digest, this version is for you. Of course, you can still add ¼ cup finely grated Parmesan if you wish. Serve with Pesto Chicken with Asparagus and Sun-Dried Tomatoes (page 111).

YIELD: 8 (2-tablespoon) servings   PREP TIME: 10 minutes
COOK TIME: none

1 cup roughly chopped fresh basil

2 cloves garlic

zest of 1 lemon

1 lemon teaspoon juice

¼ cup toasted pine nuts

¼ cup extra-virgin olive oil

sea salt

freshly ground pepper

Combine the basil, garlic, lemon zest and juice, pine nuts, and olive oil in a blender. Puree until smooth. Season to taste with salt and pepper. Store in a covered container in the refrigerator for up to 5 days or in the freezer for 1 month.

GLUTEN FREE • VEGETARIAN • DAIRY FREE • LOW CALORIE

Nutrition Facts (amount per serving)	
Calories	91
Fat	10 g
Protein	1 g
Carbohydrate	1 g
Fiber	0.4 g

MARINARA SAUCE

Most commercially prepared marinara sauces are loaded with sugar while boasting that they're low in fat. We're looking for the opposite combination in our marinara sauce. Here's a simple homemade variety you can use to top zucchini noodles, or alongside any of the calzone or pizza recipes in this book.

YIELD: 8 (½-cup) servings   PREP TIME: 5 minutes
COOK TIME: 15 minutes

¼ cup olive oil

½ cup minced onion

2 teaspoons minced garlic

1 (15-ounce) can diced plum tomatoes

1 (15-ounce) can tomato sauce

2 tablespoons roughly chopped fresh basil

sea salt

freshly ground pepper

1. Heat the olive oil in a medium saucepan and cook the onion with a generous pinch of salt until soft, about 10 minutes. Add the garlic and cook for another minute.

2. Add the diced tomatoes, tomato sauce, and basil to the pan and bring to a gentle simmer. Cook for about 5 minutes to allow the flavors to come together. Season with salt and pepper.

GLUTEN FREE · VEGETARIAN · DAIRY FREE · LOW CALORIE

Nutrition Facts
(amount per serving)

Calories	92
Fat	7 g
Protein	1 g
Carbohydrate	6 g
Fiber	1.5 g

SHEET PAN **KETOGENIC**

ENCHILADA SAUCE

Sometimes I try store-bought enchilada sauces, but this is the sauce I come back to again and again. It is smoky, sweet, spicy, and perfect for ladling over Chicken Enchilada Zucchini Boats (page 100).

YIELD: 8 (¼-cup) servings   PREP TIME: 5 minutes
COOK TIME: 10 to 15 minutes

2 tablespoons canola oil

½ cup minced yellow onion

2 cloves garlic, minced

1 (15-ounce) can tomato sauce

1 tablespoon smoked paprika

2 teaspoons ground cumin

1 teaspoon ground chipotle

¼ teaspoon ground cayenne pepper

sea salt

freshly ground pepper

1. Heat the canola oil in a small saucepan over medium heat. Add the onion, garlic, and a pinch of sea salt. Cook for 5 to 10 minutes until the onion is soft.

2. Add the tomato sauce, paprika, cumin, chipotle, and cayenne.

3. Simmer for 5 minutes. Season to taste with salt and pepper.

GLUTEN FREE ▪ VEGETARIAN ▪ DAIRY FREE ▪ LOW CALORIE

Nutrition Facts	
(amount per serving)	
Calories	52
Fat	4 g
Protein	1 g
Carbohydrate	5 g
Fiber	1 g

BARBECUE SAUCE

This smoky, sweet, and super-savory barbecue sauce is lightly sweetened with stevia. Serve with Slow-Roasted Barbecue Ribs (page 132) or Cowboy Meatballs (page 166).

YIELD: 6 (2-tablespoon) servings   PREP TIME: 5 minutes
COOK TIME: 25 to 30 minutes

1 cup apple cider vinegar

¼ cup low-sugar ketchup

½ teaspoon garlic powder

½ teaspoon onion powder

1 teaspoon smoked paprika

¼ teaspoon ground cumin

¼ teaspoon sea salt

2 to 3 drops liquid stevia

1. Place the apple cider vinegar, ketchup, garlic powder, onion powder, smoked paprika, cumin, and sea salt in a medium saucepan. Bring to a simmer and cook for 25 to 30 minutes until reduced to about ¾ cup.

2. Stir in the liquid stevia, adding more to taste.

3. Store in a covered container in the refrigerator for up to 1 week.

GLUTEN FREE ▪ VEGETARIAN ▪ DAIRY FREE ▪ LOW CALORIE

Nutrition Facts	
(amount per serving)	
Calories	16
Fat	0 g
Protein	0 g
Carbohydrate	4 g
Fiber	0.2 g

BACON MUSTARD CREAM SAUCE

This rich, flavorful sauce combines smoky bacon, spicy garlic, and savory Dijon mustard for a delicious cream sauce. Use it to slather over roasted chicken or baked salmon. Prepare it just before serving or store in a covered container for up to 3 days.

YIELD: 4 (2-tablespoon) servings   PREP TIME: 5 minutes
COOK TIME: 20 minutes

1 slice thick-cut applewood-smoked bacon, finely diced

1 teaspoon minced garlic

2 tablespoons minced shallots

1 teaspoon minced fresh thyme

1 teaspoon Dijon mustard

½ cup heavy cream

sea salt

freshly ground black pepper

1. Cook the bacon in a small saucepan over medium-low heat until most of the fat is rendered, about 10 minutes.

2. Add the garlic, shallots, and thyme to the pan and cook until the shallots are softened, about 5 minutes.

3. Add the Dijon and heavy cream and bring to a gentle simmer for 5 minutes to thicken and infuse the cream with flavor. Season to taste with salt and pepper.

GLUTEN FREE • LOW CALORIE

Nutrition Facts	
(amount per serving)	
Calories	132
Fat	13 g
Protein	2 g
Carbohydrate	2 g
Fiber	0.1 g

TERIYAKI SAUCE

Most store-bought teriyaki sauces rely on copious amounts of brown sugar or high-fructose corn syrup to sweeten them. This version uses liquid stevia. You can opt for another calorie-free sweetener if you prefer.

YIELD: 8 (2-tablespoon) servings   PREP TIME: 5 minutes
COOK TIME: 7 minutes

1 teaspoon minced garlic

1 teaspoon minced ginger

½ cup low-sodium soy sauce

½ cup plus 1 tablespoon water, divided

2 tablespoons rice wine vinegar

4 to 5 drops liquid stevia, or to taste

1 teaspoon cornstarch

1. Place the garlic, ginger, soy sauce, ½ cup water, rice wine vinegar, and stevia in a small saucepan. Bring to a simmer over medium-low heat and cook for 5 minutes to infuse the sauce with flavor.

2. Make a slurry with the remaining 1 tablespoon of water and 1 teaspoon of cornstarch, mixing until dissolved. Pour this into the teriyaki sauce and cook just until thickened, about 2 minutes more.

3. Use immediately or store in a covered container in the refrigerator for up to 3 days.

GLUTEN FREE · VEGETARIAN · DAIRY FREE · LOW CALORIE

Nutrition Facts	
(amount per serving)	
Calories	26
Fat	0 g
Protein	2 g
Carbohydrate	3 g
Fiber	0.1 g

THAI CHILI SAUCE

Most Thai chili sauces are loaded with sugar. This version is lightly sweetened with stevia instead. Serve with Coconut Shrimp (page 48) or the Vietnamese Pork Meatball Lettuce Wraps (page 144).

YIELD: 6 (2-tablespoon) servings   PREP TIME: 5 minutes
COOK TIME: 5 minutes

2 tablespoons lime juice

2 tablespoons fish sauce

2 tablespoons rice wine vinegar

¼ cup plus 1 tablespoon water, divided

1 teaspoon minced ginger

½ teaspoon minced garlic

generous pinch red chile flakes

4 to 6 drops liquid stevia, or to taste

1 teaspoon cornstarch

1. Combine the lime juice, fish sauce, rice wine vinegar, ¼ cup water, ginger, garlic, and red chile flakes in a small saucepan over medium heat. Bring to a simmer.

2. Stir in the stevia.

3. Stir the cornstarch into the remaining tablespoon of water and pour it into the sauce. Cook just until thickened, about 1 more minute.

GLUTEN FREE · DAIRY FREE · LOW CALORIE

Nutrition Facts	
(amount per serving)	
Calories	6
Fat	0 g
Protein	0 g
Carbohydrate	1 g
Fiber	0 g

SPICY PEANUT SAUCE

This spicy Asian-fusion sauce is delicious served with lettuce cups or drizzled over a crunchy salad. For a thinner consistency, add ¼ to ½ cup of water to the sauce. To make the sauce gluten-free, use gluten-free soy sauce.

YIELD: 10 (2-tablespoon) servings   PREP TIME: 5 minutes
COOK TIME: none

1 teaspoon minced ginger

1 teaspoon minced garlic

pinch red chile flakes

1 tablespoon toasted sesame oil

2 tablespoons reduced-sodium soy sauce

1 tablespoon fresh lime juice

1 cup creamy natural peanut butter

2 to 3 drops liquid stevia (optional)

1. Combine all of the ingredients in a blender and puree until smooth.

2. Store in a covered container in the refrigerator for up to 3 days.

GLUTEN FREE • VEGETARIAN • DAIRY FREE • LOW CALORIE

Nutrition Facts	
(amount per serving)	
Calories	167
Fat	14 g
Protein	7 g
Carbohydrate	6 g
Fiber	2 g

SAVOY CABBAGE AND ALMOND SLAW

This bright, tangy salad is delicious with Citrus and Herb Marinated Pork Shoulder (page 134).

YIELD: 4 servings   PREP TIME: 5 minutes   COOK TIME: none

1 scallion, thinly sliced

4 cups shredded Savoy cabbage

2 tablespoons minced fresh cilantro

2 tablespoons minced fresh mint

3 tablespoons canola oil

1 tablespoon toasted sesame oil

2 tablespoons lime juice

½ cup toasted almond slices

1. Toss the scallion, cabbage, cilantro, and mint in a large serving bowl.

2. In a separate container, whisk the canola oil, sesame oil, and lime juice, and season with salt and pepper.

3. Pour the dressing over the salad and stir gently to mix. Top with the toasted almond slices.

GLUTEN FREE · VEGETARIAN · DAIRY FREE · LOW CALORIE

Nutrition Facts	
(amount per serving)	
Calories	249
Fat	23 g
Protein	5 g
Carbohydrate	8 g
Fiber	3.8 g

SPICY KALE SALAD

This is my go-to kale salad. It works well as a side dish for so many meaty main dishes, offering brightness in flavor and a textural contrast. By massaging the kale leaves with salt and oil, the greens release some of their moisture, become softer, and have a heavier mouthfeel than most salads, which can sometimes feel like eating fluff. When I want a little more substance, I add avocado, shaved fennel, or toasted sunflower seeds, but these are optional.

YIELD: 4 servings   PREP TIME: 5 minutes   COOK TIME: none

1 bunch kale, stems removed

1 teaspoon pureed garlic

pinch red chile flakes

3 tablespoons extra-virgin olive oil

2 teaspoons white wine vinegar

sea salt

Optional add-ins:

1 avocado, diced

½ fennel bulb, thinly sliced with a vegetable peeler

¼ cup toasted sunflower seeds

1. Slice the kale leaves into bite-size pieces. Place them in a medium bowl and sprinkle with a generous pinch of sea salt. Add the garlic and red chile flakes.

2. Drizzle the olive oil over the kale, and with clean hands, massage the kale leaves gently, working the salt and oil into the leaves until they become soft and deepen in color.

3. Season with the white wine vinegar and toss to mix. Sprinkle with avocado, fennel, and sunflower seeds, if using, and toss gently to mix. Serve immediately.

GLUTEN FREE ▪ VEGETARIAN ▪ DAIRY FREE ▪ LOW CALORIE

Nutrition Facts	
(amount per serving)	
Calories	110
Fat	10 g
Protein	1 g
Carbohydrate	4 g
Fiber	1.3 g

CAULIFLOWER RICE

We all know that white rice is packed with carbs, but it's pretty jaw dropping when you read the nutrition label—45 grams per cup. Yikes! This cauliflower rice has a similar texture to white rice with a fraction of the carbs. It serves as the perfect backdrop for a wide array of dishes, especially Moroccan Chicken Tagine (page 106), or jazz it up with herbs, nuts, and whatever protein you prefer for an entree salad.

YIELD: 4 (1-cup) servings   PREP TIME: 5 minutes   COOK TIME: 5 minutes

1 medium head cauliflower, broken into florets

1 tablespoon canola oil

sea salt

1. Place the cauliflower florets into a food processor and pulse until it is coarsely ground, about the texture of white rice.

2. Squeeze the cauliflower a handful at a time to remove some of the moisture.

3. Heat a large skillet over medium-high heat. Add the canola oil and heat for 30 seconds, coating the bottom of the pan. Add the cauliflower and stir-fry for about 5 minutes until just heated through. Season with salt and serve immediately.

GLUTEN FREE ▪ VEGETARIAN ▪ DAIRY FREE ▪ LOW CALORIE

Nutrition Facts	
(amount per serving)	
Calories	67
Fat	4 g
Protein	3 g
Carbohydrate	8 g
Fiber	3.6 g

MASHED CAULIFLOWER

Mashed potatoes have met their match in this creamy, low-carb puree. It's delicious with Prime Rib Roast (page 176) and Slow-Roasted Barbecue Ribs (page 132), or wherever you usually enjoy mashed potatoes.

YIELD: 8 (½-cup) servings   PREP TIME: 5 minutes
COOK TIME: 10 minutes

1 medium head cauliflower, broken into florets

1 cup heavy cream

2 cloves garlic, smashed

1 sprig thyme

1 stick (½ cup) butter

sea salt

1. Place the cauliflower into a steamer basket in a medium pot with about 1 inch of water in it. Steam for about 10 minutes or until tender.

2. Meanwhile, bring the heavy cream to a simmer in a small skillet with the garlic and thyme. Remove the pan from the heat and allow to steep while the cauliflower cooks. Remove the garlic and thyme.

3. Transfer the cauliflower and hot cream to a blender in batches and puree until smooth.

4. Fold in the butter and season to taste with salt.

GLUTEN FREE · VEGETARIAN · LOW CALORIE

Nutrition Facts	
(amount per serving)	
Calories	222
Fat	23 g
Protein	2 g
Carbohydrate	5 g
Fiber	1.8 g

Conversions

Volume Conversions		
U.S.	U.S. equivalent	Metric
1 tablespoon (3 teaspoons)	½ fluid ounce	15 milliliters
¼ cup	2 fluid ounces	60 milliliters
⅓ cup	3 fluid ounces	90 milliliters
½ cup	4 fluid ounces	120 milliliters
⅔ cup	5 fluid ounces	150 milliliters
¾ cup	6 fluid ounces	180 milliliters
1 cup	8 fluid ounces	240 milliliters
2 cups	16 fluid ounces	480 milliliters

Temperature Conversions	
Fahrenheit (°F)	Celsius (°C)
125°F	50°C
150°F	65°C
175°F	80°C
200°F	95°C
225°F	110°C
250°F	120°C
275°F	135°C
300°F	150°C
325°F	165°C
350°F	175°C
375°F	190°C
400°F	200°C
425°F	220°C
450°F	230°C

Weight Conversions	
U.S.	Metric
½ ounce	15 grams
1 ounce	30 grams
2 ounces	60 grams
¼ pound	115 grams
⅓ pound	150 grams
½ pound	225 grams
¾ pound	350 grams
1 pound	450 grams

About the Author

Pamela Ellgen is a food blogger and cookbook author of *Sheet Pan Paleo*, *Cast Iron Paleo*, *The Microbiome Cookbook*, *Soup & Comfort*, and *Modern Family Table*. She also writes on fitness and nutrition, and her work has appeared on LIVESTRONG, Spinning.com, and the *Huffington Post*. When she's not in the kitchen, Pamela enjoys surfing, practicing yoga, and playing with her kids. She lives in California with her husband and two children.